The Breastfeeding Recipe Book

Hannah Crawford

ISBN-13: 978-1544293158

ISBN-10: 1544293151

Penguinies@outlook.com

I would like to dedicate this book to Bradley, for blessing me with our beautiful baby boy and giving me the inspiration to write this book. I will love you always & forever.

Contents

Introduction

I decided to write this breastfeeding book as I felt that there was not enough information, help or advice available for new mothers who intend to breastfeed their newborn babies. During both of my pregnancies, I was given absolutely no information about breastfeeding, even though I had mentioned it at every midwife, doctor and hospital appointment that I had attended. I wasn't provided with even the basic of information such as wired bras, breast pumps, night feeds, healthy diet and the health benefits of breastfeeding.

Consequently, I spent numerous hours carrying out my research during my pregnancy and after the birth of my son, to ensure that I had equipped myself with enough knowledge about breastfeeding. In addition to studying healthy diets and receiving a diploma in Human Nutrition.

Experts recommend that mothers should exclusively breastfeed their babies until they are six months old. However, new statistics show that the number of new mothers who have chosen to breastfeed their babies has fallen for the first time in nearly a decade. The statistics also reveal that over 300,000 mothers in Britain were not breastfeeding their babies at all by the time it came to their child's six and eight-week check-ups.

Some new mothers may feel too worried or unsupported to even try breastfeeding due to the lack of information and encouragement that is currently being provided. I found that I was given far more information about formula milk and how to sterilise bottles, than I ever was about breastfeeding, even though I had informed the midwives from day one that I intended to breastfeed both of my children. I believe that it is the mothers personal choice to decide whether or not if she wants to breastfeed her newborn baby, nonetheless, how can a mother indeed make a certain decision is she has not being provided with enough information about breastfeeding in the first place?

There is an extensive range of promotions for infant formula milk on television and radio advertisements, magazine promotions and internet campaigns that are shown every single day. One of the major companies who manufacture formula milk had one of their advertisements banned for claiming that their formula milk is the next best thing to breast milk. The advertisement went on to claim that the formula milk provided calcium for 'strong bones' and iron for 'brain development.' The advertisement was officially banned for exaggerating the product's health benefits. The Advertising Standards Authority stated that the formula milk company had misrepresented the health effects of their product. Since 2007, companies have been banned from promoting powdered milk for babies under the age of six months, as part of the Governments 'Breast is Best' campaign.

Why do we see more adverts and promotions in the media for formula milk than we do for breastfeeding? I rarely see breastfeeding in the media, and whenever I do it is always depicted in a negative light, such as, 'Woman kicked out of a shop for breastfeeding in public,' 'Woman asked to leave restaurant for breastfeeding her infant in public.' These negative headlines are not encouraging for new mothers, if anything these stories are put out there in the media to make new mothers feel nervous and insecure about breastfeeding, particularly in public. We are made to believe that this is how a large majority of the public feel about breastfeeding, which is far from true.

From pregnancy, I always intended to do the natural thing and give both of my children the best start in life, by providing them with the healthiest start possible. I spent numerous hours carrying out research on breastfeeding and studying for my diploma in Human Nutrition to prepare myself for my baby's arrival. I researched breastfeeding tips, health benefits, NHS advice, the best breastfeeding diets and foods to eat, as well as comparing different countries attitudes, and information about breastfeeding.

This information helped me to prepare and breastfeed my children for the first years of their lives. This is the reason why I feel so passionate about writing this book. I hope to help all new mothers out there who are considering and have started breastfeeding their babies.

Breastfeeding is inexpensive and can save you money over the months and years. Not only does breastfeeding benefit your child's health, but it also has health benefits for the mothers to such as weight loss. Eating healthy is important for both the mother and the baby while nursing. However, nobody said you have to deprive yourself of treats and sweets. This book is jam packed full of 180 recipes to help boost your milk supply and energy levels as well as keeping you and your baby nutritiously healthy.

I hope you enjoy reading this breastfeeding recipe book and find the information as helpful as I do and the food just as delicious.

Is Breast Best?

We are constantly having infant formula milk promoted to us, and rarely see breastfeeding campaigns or advertisements in the media. So is breast really best? Or is formula milk more beneficial for babies?

Breast milk is the most natural and healthiest way to feed your baby. Despite the formula advertisements, breastmilk is a complete food which contains at least four-hundred nutrients for your baby. Vitamins and minerals such as iron, zinc, and calcium are better absorbed in breast milk compared to formula milk. Breast milk adjusts to infant's needs; it is rich in brain building omega 3's, it is rich in cholesterol, contains fat and is nearly completely absorbed. Formula milk does not adjust to an infant's needs, and it is not completely absorbed. Breast milk also contains hormone and disease fighting compounds that your baby can not get in infant formula milk. The hormones contribute to your babies well-being and biochemical balance.

Breastmilk is the only food naturally designed for your baby, and it contains everything your child needs for around the first six months of their lives. Proteins in breast milk are rich in brain and body building protein components, as well as being easily digestible whey. Formula milk is harder to digest causing curds. Formula milk is low or deficient in some brain and body building proteins, and deficient in growth factors. Breast milk proteins also contain sleep-inducing proteins which are absent in formula milk. Breast milk is rich in lactose which is missing in some formula milk altogether. Lactose is an important carbohydrate for brain development.

Formula milk cannot give your baby the same ingredients or provide the same protection as breast milk can. Breastfeeding your baby breast milk for the first six months is extremely beneficial for your infant. One of the benefits is that it can improve your child's cognitive development. Therefore, breastfeeding your baby could make them more intelligent. Studies show that the level of lactose in the milk of a species correlates with the size of the brain of that species. Research has shown that babies who were born prematurely and fed breast milk have higher IQ's, working memory and motor functions; they are also at a lower risk of having necrotizing enterocolitis.

Breast milk contains the flavors of the mother's diet, which can influence the tastes of your child to family foods, whereas formula milk always tastes the same.

Another benefit of breastfeeding your baby from birth is that your child is less likely to become ill in their first year of life. Breast milk is rich in living white blood cells, which is absent in formula milk. While I was breastfeeding both of my sons they never once suffered from colic, and never fell ill while I was breastfeeding them. My eldest son's first illness and trip to the doctors was with an ear infection that he fell ill with a month after I had stopped breastfeeding him. Breastfeeding can help your baby to fend off other illnesses such as ear infections, bronchiolitis, gastroenteritis, and pneumonia.

Scientific research has also shown that babies who are exclusively breastfed for the first 3-4 months of their lives are less likely to get;

- Severe diarrhea

- Chest infections

- Middle ear infections

- Urine infections

- Eczema

- Diabetes as a child

Breastfeeding provides protections against numerous diseases and disorders and the advantages last well into childhood. Breastfed babies also have a lower rate of severe eczema, than babies who were formula fed. This is because breastmilk can help to delay your child's first development of eczema.

Breastfeeding helps to build a strong bond between mother and baby, both physically and emotionally. Breastfeeding benefits both the mother and baby; although it is not always easy breastfeeding is a skill that has to be learned in the days following the birth of your baby. Breastfeeding can assist new mothers in losing the baby weight that they may have gained during pregnancy. Importantly, breastfeeding encourages the mother's stomach to contract back to normal after she has given birth. Breastfeeding can reduce the mother's risk of developing type 2 diabetes. It can also lower the mother's risk of breast cancer, and protect against ovarian cancer before the menopause.

You can breastfeed directly from the breast or express and give the breastmilk to your baby in a bottle. Some mothers choose to combine breast milk and formula feeding to suit their personal circumstances. Surgery or disease may affect the necessary underlying structures. However, very few women are incapable of breastfeeding. A woman's ability to produce milk is not affected by her breast size or nipple shape.

Babies are born with inbuilt reflexes that ensure they can locate, latch onto and suck from a breast. Albeit, some mothers may need some help with the technique. There is no preparation time and no need for sterilisation unless you choose to feed your baby breast milk in a bottle. Breast milk is always delivered at exactly the right temperature. Breastmilk is the only food specifically made for human babies, and it contains everything your baby needs for around the first six months of their lives.

Colostrum

All pregnant women make milk for their baby which is available at birth.

The first milk that your body will produce is called colostrum, it is extremely concentrated and a creamy yellow colour. As the colostrum is highly concentrated, babies only need a small amount for each feed, typically a teaspoon size. Colostrum is sometimes referred to as being 'liquid gold' and is full of germ-fighting antibodies that can help to protect your baby against infections that you may have had in the past.

All babies have different feeding habits and individual needs. Your baby may want to feed every hour like my son. This usually happens in the very beginning until your milk comes in and your baby then starts to have bigger feeds and will wait longer between each feed. The first few breastfeeds will help to protect your baby's guts from germs as well as reducing the chances of developing allergies when they get older.

The more frequently you breastfeed, the more milk your body will produce. The milk will look thin compared to the colostrum although it will soon become creamer as your baby feeds.

The let-down reflex

Let down reflex is caused when your baby's suckling causes the milk stored inside of your breasts to be squeezed down ducts, towards your nipples. Some mothers feel nothing at all when this happens, and some mothers feel a tingling sensation. Your baby will respond by changing to deep rhythmic swallows as the milk flows.

Babies will often pause after the initial quick sucks. They do this because they are waiting for more milk to be delivered from your breast. If it seems like your baby has fallen to sleep before they have got to the deep swallowing stage, you should check to see if they are effectively attached to the breast.

Your breasts will respond to your baby's cries and your baby's needs. They may also respond to a warm bath or a warm shower. My breasts did not respond to a warm bath. However, they would always respond to a hot shower. Don't panic it is completely normal. You may also notice that your breasts occasionally respond to another babies crying, again this is absolutely normal and nothing to worry about.

Producing more milk

I remember being anxious when my son was born, during the first 4-5 days because I thought that I wasn't producing enough milk. This can be very upsetting and stressful for any new mother, but it really isn't anything to panic about. I was advised by my midwife to use my breast pump whenever my son wasn't feeding to encourage the milk flow, and sure enough, it worked. You may feel your breasts feeling a lot fuller and warmer immediately after the birth or a few days after giving birth. People refer to this as 'milk coming in.'

As every baby has different feeding needs, your milk will vary to suit your own baby's needs. Every time you baby feeds your body will prepare itself to make the next feed. The amount of milk you will produce depends on how often and how long your baby feeds for.

One of the most important things to know about breastfeeding, which I was not informed about, was to feed throughout the night, even if your baby does not wake for a feed. This is important as it can increase or decrease your milk flow. Feeding your baby at night or pumping your breast milk at night is important as your body produces more hormones which increase your milk supply. This can become extremely tiring, and occasionally you may need some support from your partner or family with the night feeds, but your body will soon get used to it.

Each baby feeds for different lengths of time. My son sometimes feeds for forty minutes, and other times he will only feed for five minutes. Let your baby decided when they have had enough.

In the first few months, it can feel like you're doing nothing but feeding your baby. This is because both of you are still getting into a routine, and your baby is growing and changing every single day. Once your baby gets into a good feeding routine, it will settle down and become a lot easier.

Losing weight while breastfeeding

One of the main reasons why I decided to write this breastfeeding recipe book was because everybody kept asking me how I had managed to lose all of my baby weight so fast, and what foods was I eating? Through eating these healthy recipes but not depriving myself of sweets and treats and doing some light exercise I managed to effortlessly lose two stone within seven weeks of giving birth to my son.

Breastfeeding helps to burn around 500 extra calories a day that is equivalent to a 5k run while you're sitting on the sofa feeding your baby. The best way to lose your pregnancy weight is to do it gradually and to never put pressure on yourself. You shouldn't try to lose weight through dieting until at least 2-3 months after your baby is born. Breastfeeding can be hard and extremely tiring at times, so eating plenty of vitamins and energy boosting foods is essential. Following a reduced-calorie diet while breastfeeding your baby could drain your energy and diminish your milk supply.

Some new mothers find that the pregnancy weight just seems to fall off while they are breastfeeding while others struggle to get back to their pre-pregnancy weight. This is because we all have different bodies, varying levels of activity, we make different food choices, and we have different metabolisms.

If you are overweight and finding it extremely hard to lose the gained pounds, you should talk to your doctor or health professional before starting on a diet.

As soon as you have given birth most of the pregnancy diet restrictions are lifted, which means you can eat blue cheese, mayonnaise, and liver pâté.

Staying hydrated is also crucial while breastfeeding. I found that I was so thirsty in the first few months of breastfeeding and I couldn't drink enough water. It is important that you listen to your body. Natural ingredients and teas can help to increase your milk supply. This is why I have included plenty of drink and ice tea recipes in this breastfeeding recipe book.

Taking care of your body by eating healthy and doing some light exercise is one the best ways of ensuring that you stay healthy and lose some pregnancy weight.

Eating a variety of foods and maintaining a balanced diet is essential for your body to repair itself after giving birth as well as providing your newborn baby with a good supply of breast milk. The nutrients will help your child to develop and grow.

A balanced diet should consist of a mix of:

- Protein – eggs, fish, meat, nuts, pulses

- Calcium – cheese, milk, yogurts

- Whole grain carbohydrates – bread, pasta, and rice

- Fruits and vegetables (at least five portions a day)

- Drink plenty of water; try to aim for 8-16 pints a day

Understanding the role that nutrition plays in our growth and development throughout life is very important. For our bodies to maintain numerous bodily functions and to provide us with energy we must consume macronutrients on a daily basis.

Micronutrients such as vitamin C, vitamin E and selenium help to prevent and delay different types of cell damage that may occur in the body. Therefore, foods containing them are extremely beneficial for a nursing mother's health.

Breastfeeding Recipe Book

Breastfeeding Recipe Book

Smoothies

Breakfast

Salads

Soups

Main Meals

Desserts

Snacks & Sides

- Homemade Peanut Butter – Page 174
- Lactation Cookies – Page 175-176
- Pineapple Cinnamon Strips – Page 177
- Stuffed Peppers – Page 178-179
- Spicy Sweet Potato Chips – Page 180
- Seasoned Yorkshire Puddings – Page 181-182
- Seasoned Vegetables – Page 183-184
- Mediterranean Vegetables – Page 185-186
- Parmesan Straws – Page 187
- Cheesy Chili Relleno Squares – Page 188
- Rosemary Roast Potatoes – Page 189-190

Bread

- Cloud Bread – Page 192
- Soda Bread – Page 193
- Garlic Bread – Page 194-195
- Sesame Seed Bread Rolls – Page 196-197
- Cheesy Garlic Bread – Page 198-199
- Focaccia with Pesto & Mozzarella – Page 200-201
- Sundried Tomato & Olive Bread – Page 202-203
- Rustic Rolls – Page 204-205

Jams

- Strawberry Jam – Page 207-208
- Raspberry Jam – Page 209
- Blackberry Jam – Page 210-211
- Plum Jam – Page 212
- Pineapple Jam - Page 213
- Peach Jam – Page 214
- Marmalade – Page 215-216

Popcorn

- Toffee Popcorn – Page 218-219
- Popcorn Balls – Page 220-221

Drinks

Homemade Cordial

Mocktails

Smoothies

Pink Oat Delight Smoothie

Ingredients

- 150ml Whole Milk
- 50g Raspberries
- 50g Oats
- 50g Banana
- 30g Pink Grapefruit
- 5g Fresh Ginger

Method

1. Place50g of raspberries, fresh or frozen and 50g of oats into a blender.
2. Peel and chop the banana, ginger, and grapefruit and then add the correct amounts to the blender.
3. Blend the ingredients for 1-2 minutes.
4. Pour 150ml of whole milk into the blender and blitz for a further 2-3 minutes.
5. Pour into a glass and serve.

*Top Tip

You can add a teaspoon of honey to sweeten up the smoothie to suit your taste.

Berry Smoothie

Ingredients

- 250g Berries Fresh/Frozen
- 250g Strawberry Yogurt
- 50ml Whole Milk
- 15g Oats
- 1 Teaspoon Honey

Method

1. Place 250g of either fresh or frozen berry's into a blender along with 250g of strawberry yogurt and 50ml of whole milk. Blend the ingredients for 1-2 minutes or until smooth.
2. Add 15g of oats and 1 teaspoon of honey to the ingredients and blitz for a further 1-2 minutes.
3. Pour the smoothie out into a glass and serve.

*Top Tip

You can add more or less honey to suit your personal taste.

Energy Smoothie

Ingredients

- 1 Ripe Banana
- 1 Handful of Spinach
- 180ml Milk

Method

1. Chop 1 ripe banana up and place the chunks in a blender.
2. Add 1 handful of washed spinach to the blender and 180ml of milk.
3. Blitz the blender for 1-2 minutes.
4. Pour into a glass and serve.

*Top Tip

You can add a teaspoon of honey to sweeten up the smoothie to suit your taste.

Banana Orange Smoothie

Ingredients
- 1 Ripe Banana
- 1 Orange
- 1 Teaspoon of Vanilla Extract
- 180ml Milk
- 120g Plain Greek Yogurt

Method

1. Chop 1 ripe banana up and place the chunks in a blender.
2. Peel 1 orange and divide it up. Add the orange segments to the blender.
3. Pour 180ml of milk and 120g of plain Greek yogurt into the blender.
4. Add 1 teaspoon of vanilla extract to the fruit.
5. Blitz the blender for 1-2 minutes.
6. Pour into a glass and serve.

*Top Tip

You can add a teaspoon of honey to sweeten up the smoothie to suit your taste.

Chocolate Peanut Butter Smoothie

Ingredients
- 1 Ripe Banana
- 180ml Milk
- 1 Tablespoon Natural Peanut Butter
- 2-3 Teaspoons Cocoa Powder

Method

1. Chop 1 ripe banana up and place the chunks in a blender.
2. Add 180ml of milk to the blender, followed by 1 tablespoon of natural peanut butter and 2-3 teaspoons of cocoa powder.
3. Blitz the blender for 1-2 minutes.
4. Pour into a glass and serve.

*Top Tip

You can add a teaspoon of honey to sweeten up the smoothie to suit your taste.

Pina Colada Smoothie

Ingredients

- 2 Ripe Bananas
- 140g Pineapple Chunks
- 1 Can of Coconut Milk

Method

1. Chop 2 ripe bananas up and place the chunks in a blender.
2. Add 140g of fresh or canned pineapple chunks to the banana.
3. Pour 1 can of coconut milk into the blender.
4. Blitz the blender for 1-2 minutes.
5. Pour into a glass and serve.

Strawberry Banana Smoothie

Ingredients
- 1 Banana
- 85g Strawberries
- 180ml Milk
- 120g Plain Greek Yogurt

Method

1. Chop 1 ripe banana up and place the chunks in a blender.
2. Add 85g of fresh or frozen strawberries to the banana.
3. Pour 180ml of milk and 120g of plain Greek Yogurt into the blender.
4. Blitz the blender for 1-2 minutes.
5. Pour into a glass and serve.

Breakfast

Berry Porridge

Ingredients
- 290ml Milk or Water
- 80g Oats
- 80g Blueberries
- 80g Raspberries
- 1-2 Teaspoons of Honey

Method

1. Add 80g of oats to a saucepan and place over a medium heat.
2. Pour in 290ml of Milk or Water and then bring to the boil, stirring frequently.
3. Simmer for a 2-3 minutes before removing the pan from the heat.

Option 1

1. Blend 80g of raspberries along with 80g of blueberries.
2. Add 1-2 teaspoons of honey and blend for one minute.
3. Pour the berry mixture into the pan of oats and stir. Simmer on a low-medium heat for 3-4 minutes.
4. Divide the porridge into two bowls and serve.

Option 2

1. Pour the porridge into two bowls and give it a quick stir.

2. Sprinkle 40g of raspberries and 40g of blueberries on top of each bowl of porridge.
3. Add one teaspoon of honey to the top of each of the fruit.
4. Serve.

*Top Tip

Add in a few almonds for extra taste and an added energy boost.

Banana Pancakes

Ingredients
- 225ml Milk
- 125g Plain Flour
- 2 Teaspoons of Baking Powder
- 2 Tablespoons of Caster Sugar
- 1 Egg
- 2 Tablespoons of Vegetable Oil
- 2 Ripe Bananas, Mashed

Method
1. Pour 125g of plain flour into a bowl. Add 2 tablespoons of caster sugar and 2 teaspoons of baking power. Mix the ingredients together.
2. In a separate bowl crack and beat 1 egg.
3. Add 2 tablespoons of vegetable oil and two mashed bananas to the egg and mix.
4. Combine the flour, caster sugar and baking powder into the banana mixture. (The mixture will be slightly lumpy.)
5. Lightly oil a frying pan or a griddle and place over a medium/high heat.
6. Scoop approximately 4 tablespoons of the batter into the hot pan. Cook for 2-3 minutes either side or until the pancakes are golden brown on both sides.
7. Serve hot.

Berry Pancakes

Ingredients
- 225ml Milk
- 125g Plain Flour
- 110g Mixed Berries (Or Berries of Your Choice.)
- 2 Teaspoons of Baking Powder
- 2 Tablespoons of Caster Sugar
- 2 Tablespoons of Vegetable Oil
- 1 Egg

Garnish
- Handful of Mixed Berries

Method

1. Pour 125g of plain flour into a bowl. Add 2 tablespoons of caster sugar and 2 teaspoons of baking power. Mix the ingredients together.
2. In a separate bowl crack and beat 1 egg.
3. Add 2 tablespoons of vegetable oil and 110g of mixed berries to the whisked egg and mix.
4. Combine the flour, caster sugar and baking powder in with the berry mixture. (The mixture will be slightly lumpy.)
5. Lightly oil a frying pan or a griddle and place over a medium/high heat.
6. Scoop approximately 4 tablespoons of the batter into the hot pan. Cook for 2-3 minutes either side or until the pancakes are golden brown on both sides.
7. Serve hot.
8. To garnish sprinkle a handful of mixed berries on top of each of the pancakes.

Turkey & Spinach Omelet

Ingredients

- 85g Deli Cut Turkey
- 40g Chopped Onion
- 30g of Baby Spinach Leafs
- 28g Grated Cheddar Cheese
- 2 Eggs

Method

1. Lightly oil a frying pan and place over a medium/high heat.
2. Crack and beat 2 eggs in a small bowl.
3. Place 40g of chopped onion, 15g of baby spinach leafs and 85g of deli cut turkey into the frying pan and cook for 5-6 minutes.
4. Beat the egg for a further minute and then pour into the pan over the ingredients. Cook each side for 3-4 minutes or until the center of the omelet begins to look dry.
5. Sprinkle 28g of grated cheddar cheese on top of the omelet along with 15g of baby spinach leafs.
6. Gently fold one edge of the omelet over so that the cheese and spinach leafs are now in the middle of the omelet. Cook for a further 1-2 minutes or until the cheese starts to melt.
7. Serve.

Bacon & Pepper Omelet

Ingredients

- 85g of Cubed or shredded Bacon
- 40g Mixed Peppers
- 40g Chopped Onion
- 28g Grated Cheddar Cheese
- 2 Eggs

Method

1. Lightly oil a frying pan and place over a medium/high heat.
2. Crack and beat 2 eggs in a small bowl.
3. Place 40g of chopped onion, 40g of mixed peppers and 85g of cubed or shredded bacon into the frying pan and cook for 6-8 minutes.
4. Beat the egg for a further minute and then pour into the pan over the ingredients. Cook each side for 3-4 minutes or until the center of the omelet begins to look dry.
5. Sprinkle 28g of grated cheddar cheese on top of the omelet.
6. Gently fold one edge of the omelet over so that the cheese is now in the middle of the omelet. Cook for a further 1-2 minutes or until the cheese starts to melt.
7. Serve.

Spinach Scrambled Eggs

Ingredients
- 45g of Baby Spinach Leafs
- 30g of Grated Cheddar Cheese.
- 2 Tablespoons of Butter
- 2 Eggs
- ½ Teaspoon of Salt
- ½ Teaspoon of Ground Black Pepper

Method

1. Crack and beat 2 eggs in a small bowl.
2. Add ½ teaspoon of salt and ½ teaspoon of ground black pepper into the eggs and whisk.
3. Add 2 tablespoons of butter to a frying pan and place over a medium heat until the butter has melted.
4. Pour the eggs into the pan and cook for 4-5 minutes. Continuously stir the eggs until curds start to form.
5. Add 45g of baby spinach leafs to the pan and cook for a further 3-4 minutes.
6. Sprinkle 30g of grated cheddar cheese onto the eggs and cook for 1-2 minutes or until the cheese begins to melt.
7. Remove the pan from the heat and serve immediately.

*Top Tip

Try eating your spinach scrambled eggs with an English muffin or a slice of whole grain bread toasted.

Baked Egg & Soldiers

Ingredients
- Rapeseed Oil
- 2 Eggs
- Pinch of Salt
- Pinch of Ground Black Pepper
- 2 Slices of Seed Wheat Bread

Method

1. Preheat the oven to 200c/ gas mark 6.
2. Lightly grease two ovenproof ramekins or two small baking dishes with rapeseed oil.
3. Crack 1 egg in each of the ramekin bowls.
4. Lightly season each of the eggs with a pinch of salt and a pinch of ground black pepper.
5. Place the ramekin bowls in the oven and bake for 8-10 minutes or until the egg whites set.
6. Cut two slices of seed wheat bread up into long strips, approximately 2.5cm wide. Butter the bread if desired.
7. Take the ramekins out of the oven and serve straight away.

*Top Tip

Baked Eggs are very versatile, try adding different ingredients to the ramekin bowls to create different flavors such as tomato, basil, spinach, turkey, ham, chives, mushrooms and smoked salmon.

Salads

Chicken & Bacon Salad

Ingredients

- 100g Crispy Lettuce
- 2 Cooked & Boneless Chicken Breasts
- 4 Rashers of Streaky Bacon Diced or Shredded
- 1 Red Onion
- 2 Tablespoons of Olive Oil
- 2 Tablespoons of White Wine Vinegar
- Pinch of Ground Black Pepper
- 5 Cherry Tomatoes
- ¼ Cucumber

Method

1. Add 4 rashers of diced or shredded streaky bacon to a lightly oiled frying pan and place over a medium/high heat. Cook for 4-6 minutes or until the bacon becomes crisp. Drain the bacon on kitchen paper.
2. Peel and dice 1 red onion and place in a bowl.
3. Add 2 tablespoons of olive oil and 2 tablespoons of white wine vinegar to the onion and stir.
4. Add 100g of washed crispy lettuce to the onion and stir.
5. Dice ¼ cucumber and chop 5 cherry tomatoes, add the ingredients to the bowl and mix together.
6. Shred 2 cooked, boneless chicken breasts and add to the salad bowl. Mix the ingredients well so that it is evenly spread out.
7. Sprinkle the bacon pieces on top of the salad and lightly season with a pinch of ground black pepper.
8. Serve.

*Top Tip

You can serve the chicken & bacon salad with some fresh crispy bread. You can also experiment with making different salad dressings to suit your taste buds such as Greek yogurt.

Feta Cheese Salad

Ingredients
- 200g Feta Cheese
- 100g Curly Leaf Lettuce
- 3 Large Tomatoes
- ½ Cucumber
- 1 Red Onion
- 1 Teaspoon of Dried Oregano
- 40g of Black Olives, Pitted
- Pinch of Salt
- Pinch of Ground Black Pepper
- 1 Teaspoon of Olive Oil

Method

1. Chop 3 large tomatoes and ½ cucumber up into small pieces and place in a salad bowl.
2. Peel and dice 1 red onion and add it to the salad bowl. Sprinkle a pinch of salt and a pinch of ground black pepper on top and mix together.
3. Add 1 teaspoon of olive oil to the ingredients and 1 teaspoon of dried oregano and lightly stir.
4. Shred or chop 100g of washed curly leaf lettuce and place it in the salad bowl. Blend all of the ingredients together so that they are evenly spread out.
5. Chop or crumble the feta cheese and sprinkle over the salad along with the black olives.
6. Serve.

*Top Tip

Allowing the salt, tomatoes, and cucumbers to marinate before adding any other oil is an essential to any good Greek salad. Try eating this salad with some freshly made bread or with some seeded wholemeal bread.

Walnut Pasta Salad

Ingredients

- 350g Fusilli Pasta
- 40g Black Olives pitted
- 1 Red Onion
- 100g Walnuts
- 220g Tomatoes
- 35ml Olive Oil
- 60g Parmesan Cheese shaved
- 30ml White Balsamic Vinegar
- 2 Stick of Celery
- Pinch of Salt
- Pinch of Ground Black Pepper

Method

1. Boil 350g of fusilli pasta in a large saucepan filled with water until al dente, then remove from the heat and drain.
2. Chop 2 sticks of washed celery into small pieces and place them in a salad bowl.
3. Peel and chop 1 red onion into little pieces and add to the salad bowl.
4. Chop 220g of tomatoes into small wedges and add them to the celery and onion.
5. Add 100g of walnuts and 40g of black olives to the salad bowl and mix together.
6. Gradually stir in all of the pasta.
7. Add 35ml of olive oil, 30ml of white balsamic vinegar, a pinch of salt and a pinch of ground black pepper to the pasta and mix well.
8. Scatter the parmesan cheese on top of the ingredients.
9. Serve.

Turkey Salad with Pitta Bread

Ingredients
- 200g Deli Turkey Breast
- 100g Cheddar Cheese
- 50g Lettuce
- 5 Cherry Tomatoes
- ¼ Cucumber
- 50g of Radishes
- 1 Stick of Celery
- A Pinch of Ground Black Pepper
- 1 Pitta Bread
- Mayonnaise, Optional

Method

1. Chop and shred 50g of lettuce and place in a salad bowl.
2. Chop ¼ cucumber and 1 stick of celery into small pieces and add to the salad bowl.
3. Slice and half five cherry tomatoes and add to the lettuce, cucumber, and celery.
4. Pour 50g of radishes, 200g of deli turkey breast, and a 100g of cheddar cheese into the ingredients and mix well.
5. Add a pinch of ground black pepper to the salad.
6. Add a dollop of mayonnaise to the ingredients (optional).
7. Toast or grill a pitta bread until slightly browned.
8. Fill 1 pita bread up with the ingredients and slice in half.
9. Serve.

Greek Salad

Ingredients

- 4 Tomatoes
- ½ Cucumber
- ½ Red Onion
- 40g Kalamata/ Black Olives
- 1 Teaspoon of dried oregano
- 85g Feta Cheese
- 3 Tablespoons of Greek Extra Virgin Olive Oil
- Pinch of Salt
- Pinch of Ground Black Pepper

Method

1. Chop 4 tomatoes, and ½ a cucumber up into small pieces and place in a salad bowl.
2. Peel and dice ½ red onion and add it to the salad bowl. Sprinkle a pinch of salt and a pinch of ground black pepper on top and mix together.
3. Add 40g of Kalamata or black olives to the salad bowl and mix together.
4. Cut 85g of feta cheese up into little cubes and add to the salad bowl.
5. Sprinkle 1 teaspoon of dried oregano over the ingredients and add 3 tablespoons of Greek extra virgin olive oil and mix together.
6. Serve.

*Top Tip

Allowing the salt, tomatoes, and cucumbers to marinate before adding any other oil is an essential to any good Greek salad. Try eating this salad with some freshly made bread or with some seeded wholemeal bread.

Tuna Salad

Ingredients
- 1 Tin of Tuna, Drained
- ½ Red Onion
- ¼ Cucumber
- 4 Tomatoes
- Fresh Coriander Leaves
- 1 Small Jalapeno Pepper
- Pinch of Salt
- Pinch of Ground Black Pepper

Method

1. Chop ½ red onion, ¼ cucumber, and 1 small jalapeno pepper up into little pieces and place in a salad bowl.
2. Chop 4 tomatoes up into small wedges and add to the onion, cucumber and jalapeno pepper.
3. Chop a small handful of fresh coriander leaves up and place them in the salad bowl.
4. Add 1 whole tin of drained tuna to the ingredients and stir well.
5. Lightly season the food with a pinch of salt and a pinch of ground black pepper.
6. Serve immediately or refrigerate until serving.

*Top Tip

You can try adding some lettuce or spinach leafs to your tuna salad.

SOUPS

Apple & Butternut Squash Soup

Ingredients
- 28g Butter
- 1 Butternut Squash
- 1 Green Apple
- 1 Carrot
- 1 Celery Stick
- 1 Onion
- 3 Cups of Chicken Stock
- 1 Cup of Water
- Pinch of Cinnamon
- Pinch of Nutmeg
- Pinch of Cayenne Pepper
- Pinch of Salt
- Pinch of Ground Black Pepper

Method

1. Place 28g of butter in a large pan and place over a medium/high heat.
2. Chop 1 onion, 1 carrot and 1 stick of celery up into small pieces and place in the frying pan to sauté for approximately 5-6 minutes.
3. Peel and chop 1 butternut squash up into small but thick pieces and discard the seeds.
4. Chop 1 green apple up into small pieces and discard any pips and the apple core.
5. Place both the butternut squash pieces and the apple pieces into the saucepan and add 1 cup of water, and 3 cups of chicken stock and bring to the boil.
6. Season the soup with a pinch of cinnamon, a pinch of nutmeg, a pinch of cayenne pepper, a pinch of salt

and a pinch of ground black pepper. Stir the ingredients together.

7.   Reduce the heat and cover the saucepan. Simmer for approximately 25-30 minutes.

8.   Remove the soup from the heat and purée in a blender or with an immersion blender.

9.   Serve hot or cold.

*Top Tip

You can garnish this soup with some fresh chives or parsley. Add some freshly made bread or some seeded wholemeal bread as a side for this dish.

Tomato & Basil Soup

Ingredients

- 200g Tomatoes
- 125ml Double Cream
- 1 Tablespoon of Butter
- 200ml Vegetable Stock
- 1 Teaspoon of Sugar
- 9 Leaves of Fresh Basil
- Pinch of Salt
- Pinch of Ground Black Pepper

Method

1. Chop 200g of Tomatoes up into small pieces and place in a large saucepan.
2. Pour 200ml of Vegetable stock into the saucepan over the tomatoes.
3. Place the pan on a medium heat and simmer for 10 minutes.
4. Add 1 teaspoon of sugar to the saucepan and 9 fresh leaves of basil. Simmer for a further 4-5 minutes.
5. Pour in 125ml of double cream and stir.
6. Add 1 tablespoon of butter to the soup and wait until all of the butter has melted before stirring.
7. Add a pinch of salt and a pinch of black pepper to the soup and stir.
8. Remove the soup from the heat and purée in a blender or with an immersion blender.
9. Serve hot or cold.

*Top Tip

Garnish your soup with a few leaves of fresh basil. Add some freshly made bread or some seeded wholemeal bread as a side for this dish.

Tomato & Roast Pepper Soup

Ingredients

- 200g Tomatoes
- 2 Red Peppers
- ½ Onion
- 2 Cloves of Garlic
- 1 Stick of Celery
- 15g Butter
- 1 Tablespoon of Olive Oil
- 1 Tablespoon Tomato Puree
- 1 Tablespoon of Sundried Tomato Paste
- ½ Teaspoon Flaked Chili
- 250ml Vegetable Stock
- Pinch of Salt
- Pinch of Ground Black Pepper

Method

1. Preheat your oven to 200c/gas mark 4.
2. Chop 200g of tomatoes, 2 red peppers, and ½ an onion up into small pieces and place on a baking tray.
3. Place 2 cloves of garlic onto the baking tray and drizzle the ingredients with 1 tablespoon of Olive Oil.
4. Place the baking tray into the oven and bake for 25-30 minutes or until the vegetables are roasted.
5. Place 15g of butter in a large saucepan and place over a medium heat until all of the butter has melted.
6. Chop 1 stick of celery up into small pieces and add to the pan of butter. Sauté the celery pieces for 4-5 minutes.
7. Add in 1 tablespoon of tomato puree to the saucepan along with 1 tablespoon of sundried tomato paste,

and ½ a teaspoon of flaked chili. Mix and blend the ingredients together.

8.   Pour 250ml of vegetable stock into the saucepan and stir well. Cook the ingredients for a further 5-6 minutes and then remove from the heat.

9.   Once the vegetables have roasted remove the baking tray from the oven.

10. Peel and chop the 2 cloves of garlic and add them to the saucepan.

11. Add the onions, red peppers and tomatoes to the saucepan and place on a low/medium heat.

12. Add a pinch of salt and a pinch of black pepper to the soup and stir well.

13. Remove the soup from the heat and purée in a blender or with an immersion blender.

14. Serve the soup hot or cold.

*Top Tip

Serve this soup with some fresh ciabatta bread.

Carrot & Coriander Soup

Ingredients
- 4 Large Carrots
- ½ Onion
- 900ml Vegetable Stock
- 1 Tablespoon of Coconut Oil
- A Large Bunch of Fresh Coriander

Method

1. Peel and chop 4 large carrots and ½ onion up into pieces.
2. Add 1 tablespoon of coconut oil to a large saucepan and place over a medium heat.
3. Place the chopped carrots and onions in the saucepan and sauté for 4-5 minutes.
4. Pour 900ml of vegetable stock into the saucepan and add in the fresh coriander. Stir the ingredients and bring the soup to the boil. Cook until the carrots are tender.
5. Remove the soup from the heat and purée in a blender or with an immersion blender.
6. Serve hot or cold.

*Top Tip

Serve this soup with some fresh crusty bread cobs.

Leek & Potato Soup

Ingredients

- 3 Leeks
- 3 Potatoes
- 1 Onion
- 1 Clove of Garlic
- 50g of Butter
- 900ml Chicken Stock
- Small Handful of Fresh Parsley
- 1 Bouquet Garni
- 1 Vegetable Stock Cube
- Pinch of Salt
- Pinch of Ground Black Pepper

Method

1. Place 50g of butter in a large saucepan, then place over a medium heat until all of the butter has melted.
2. Peel and chop 1 clove of garlic and 1 onion up into small pieces add to the saucepan of melted butter. Sauté the garlic and onions for 4-5 minutes.
3. Pour 900ml of chicken stock into the pan and add a small handful of fresh parsley, 1 bouquet garni, and 1vegetable stock cube. Mix the ingredients together.
4. Chop 3 leeks and 3 potatoes up into small chunks and add to the saucepan.
5. Stir the ingredients together and bring the soup to the boil. Simmer for approximately 25 minutes.
6. Remove the bouquet garni and season the soup with a pinch of salt and a pinch of ground black pepper.
7. Remove the soup from the heat and purée in a blender or with an immersion blender.
8. Serve the soup hot.

*Top Tip

If the soup becomes too thin and watery add some cornflour to the thicken the soup up.

Vegetable Soup

Ingredients
- 250g Raw Vegetables of your Choice
- 300g Potatoes
- 1 Tablespoon Rapeseed Oil
- 700ml Stock
- Pinch of Salt
- Pinch of Ground Black Pepper

Method

1. Peel and chop 250g of your chosen raw vegetables into small chunks.
2. Add 1 tablespoon of rapeseed oil to a frying pan or wok and place over a medium-high heat.
3. Place the vegetables in the frying pan and fry.
4. Peel and cube 300g of potatoes and add to the frying pan. Fry until the potatoes begin to soften.
5. Pour in 700ml of stock and simmer for 15 minutes or until the vegetables are tender.
6. Season the soup with a pinch of salt and a pinch of ground black pepper.
7. Remove the soup from the heat and purée in a blender or with an immersion blender.
8. Serve the soup hot.

*Top Tip

Serve the soup with a dollop of crème Fraiche and some fresh herbs.

Main Meals

Chicken Wrap

Ingredients

- 125g Chicken Breast
- 1 Tablespoon of Rapeseed Oil
- 1 Teaspoon of Chicken Seasoning
- ½ Teaspoon of Cayenne Pepper
- ¼ Cucumber
- 1 Tablespoon of Mayonnaise
- 1 Tortilla
- 90g Crunchy Lettuce
- 1 Tomato
- ¼ Red Pepper

Method

1. Cut 125g of boneless and skinless chicken breast up into long strips.
2. Add 1 teaspoon of chicken seasoning and ½ a teaspoon of cayenne pepper to a small bowl. Stir in the raw chicken strips and mix together, ensuring all of the chicken strips are covered in seasoning.
3. Heat 1 tablespoon of rapeseed oil in a frying pan and place over a medium/high heat.
4. Add the chicken strips to the frying pan and cook for approximately 10 minutes, or until the chicken pieces turn golden. Reduce the heat to low and simmer for a further five minutes.
5. Chop ¼ cucumber, 1 tomato, and ¼ red pepper up into small pieces and place in a small salad bowl.
6. Shred and chop 90g of crunchy lettuce and add to the salad bowl.
7. Add 1 Tablespoon of mayonnaise to the salad bowl and mix the ingredients together.

8. Place 1 tortilla on a microwavable plate and heat in the microwave for 15-20 seconds.

9. Remove the tortilla from the microwave and add an even layer of ingredients from the salad bowl.

10. Add a layer of chicken strips to the tortilla and top with a small layer of salad ingredients.

11. Fold the bottom of the tortilla and start rolling the tortilla up. When the tortilla is half rolled, fold the top of the tortilla down to enclose the filling and continue to roll the tortilla up to make a compact wrap.

12. Serve.

*Top Tip

This chicken wrap tastes nice hot or cold. To eat it cold store in the refrigerator until ready to eat. You could also try serving this chicken wrap with a small side of nachos.

Fennel & Red Onion Quiche

Ingredients
- 2 Fennel Bulbs
- 2 Red Onions
- 2 Red Chili's
- 1 Tablespoon of Fennel Seeds
- 1 Packet of Ready-rolled Shortcrust Pastry
- 1 Teaspoon of Butter
- 200ml Single Cream
- 150g Goats Cheese
- 2 Eggs
- 2 Tablespoons of Rapeseed Oil
- Salt
- Ground Black Pepper

Method

1. Preheat the oven to $180°$C/ Gas mark 4.
2. Peel 2 red onions and cut them into thin slices.
3. Heat 2 tablespoons of rapeseed oil in a frying pan and place over a medium/high heat.
4. Add the onions to the frying pan and cook for 3-4 minutes.
5. Cut 2 fennel bulbs into chunks. Discard the green leafy bits.
6. Add the fennel to the frying pan of onions. Season with a pinch of salt and a pinch of ground black pepper. Fry the ingredients for another 5 minutes.
7. Chop 2 red chili's into small pieces and remove any seeds.
8. Add the chili pieces to the frying pan and sprinkle the ingredients with 1 tablespoon of fennel seeds. Stir and set aside.

9. Grease your quiche dish with 1 teaspoon of butter (more if required).
10. Roll out the shortcrust pastry and fit it into your quiche dish. Using a knife, cut around the top of your dish.
11. Pour and spread the red onion, fennel, chili peppers, and fennel seeds evenly into the quiche dish.
12. Crack 2 eggs into a bowl and whisk.
13. Add 200ml of single cream to the eggs and stir well. Season generously with salt and pepper.
14. Pour the cream mixture over the vegetables in the quiche dish.
15. Crumble 150g of goat's cheese over the quiche.
16. Place the quiche in the oven and bake for approximately 45-50 minutes.
17. Serve hot or cold.

*Top Tip

Sprinkle the top of the quiche with fresh tarragon before serving. This fennel & red onion quiche tastes nice hot or cold with a side of salad.

Moussaka

Ingredients
- 600g Lamb Mince Meat
- 400g of Chopped Tomatoes/ Tomato Passata
- 600g Lamb Mince Meat
- 500g Potatoes
- 400g of Chopped Tomatoes/ Tomato Passata
- 2 Aubergines
- 2 Teaspoons of Rapeseed Oil
- 2 Cloves of Garlic
- 1 Tablespoon of Cinnamon
- 1 Teaspoon of Dried Oregano
- 1 Large Onion
- 1 Bay Leaf
- 1 Teaspoon of Ground Black Pepper
- 1 Tablespoon of Salt.

For the Béchamel Sauce
- 400ml Whole Milk
- 50g Butter
- 50g Plain White Flour
- 35g Grated Parmesan or Mozzarella Cheese.
- 1 Teaspoon of Nutmeg (Grated/ Dried)
- 1 Egg

Method

1. Chop 2 aubergines into 1 cm thick slices. Place the aubergines in a large mixing bowl and sprinkle with 1 tablespoon of salt.
2. Fill the bowl with fresh cold water and then place a plate or a heavy weight down on top of the aubergines and leave to soak for 40-60 minutes.
3. Peel and chop 1 large onion up into diced pieces.

4. Chop 2 cloves of garlic up into small pieces.
5. Add 600g of lamb mincemeat to a large frying pan and place over a medium/high heat. Cook for approximately 8-10 minutes, or until all of the mince has browned.
6. Once the mince has browned add the chopped onions, garlic, oregano, bay leaf, black pepper and cinnamon to the frying pan and stir well.
7. Stir in 400g of chopped tomatoes/ tomato passata into the frying pan.
8. Reduce the heat to low and cover the pan with a lid. Simmer the ingredients for 30 minutes, occasionally stirring until the lamb is tender and the sauce has thickened.
9. Rinse the aubergines in fresh cold water. Place the aubergines slices on top of some clean kitchen paper and dry.
10. In a clean frying pan heat 2 tablespoons of rapeseed oil. Add the aubergine slices and fry for 2-3 minutes on each side. Remove the aubergines from the frying pan and dry on some fresh kitchen paper.
11. Preheat the oven to 180°c/ Gas mark 4.
12. Peel 500g of potatoes and cut them into 1cm slices. Boil the potatoes in a pan of boiling water for 5-10 minutes.
13. Drain the potatoes in a colander and rinse with fresh cold water.
14. With a large spoon add a layer of the meat sauce to an ovenproof dish. Cover the meat with a layer of aubergines and then add a layer of potatoes. Repeat this process two more times, or until all of the ingredients have filled the oven proof dish.
15. In a small saucepan melt 50g of butter on a low heat.
16. Gradually stir in 50g of plain white flour.
17. Gradually add in 400ml of whole milk and stir well. Once the sauce has smoothed and thickened add 1 teaspoon of dried/grated nutmeg and half of the

parmesan or mozzarella cheese. Simmer on a low heat and gently stir for 5 minutes.

18. Season the béchamel sauce to taste with a salt and pepper.
19. Remove the saucepan from the heat and beat in the egg.
20. Pour the béchamel sauce over the Moussaka so that it covers all of the ingredients. Make sure the sauce is thick and spread out evenly.
21. Sprinkle the top of the sauce with the remaining cheese.
22. Bake in the oven for 45-50 minutes, or until the moussaka turns golden brown and crispy.

Fish Cakes

Ingredients
- 450g of Mixed Frozen Cod, Haddock & Salmon
- 450g of Potatoes
- 2 Tablespoons of Chopped Fresh Parsley
- 1 Egg
- Rapeseed oil
- Salt
- Pinch of Ground Black Pepper

Method

1. Preheat the oven to 190°C/ Gas Mark 5.
2. Fill a saucepan up with cold water and add a teaspoon of salt. Place the saucepan over a medium/high heat and bring to the boil.
3. Peel and chop 450g of potatoes into chunks.
4. Once the water has boiled, add the potatoes to the saucepan and cook for 15 minutes, or until tender.
5. Drain the potatoes in a colander and then return to the saucepan. Mash the potatoes with a potato masher until smooth, and all of the lumps have disappeared. Leave the potato to one side.
6. Place the frozen cod, haddock, and salmon on a roasting tray and cook in the oven for 12-15 minutes.
7. Once the fish has been removed from the oven and has cooled down, remove the skin and any bones.
8. Flake the fish into large chunks and place in the saucepan with the mashed potatoes.
9. Add 1 egg and 2 tablespoons of chopped fresh parsley into the mashed potato. Mix the ingredients together until they are well combined.

10. Season with a pinch of salt and a pinch of ground black pepper.
11. Shape the potato mixture into 8-10 patties. (Depending on how large or small you want your fishcakes to be you can make more or less).
12. Place the fishcakes in the refrigerator and leave for one hour.
13. Pour some rapeseed oil into a frying pan and place over a medium/high heat.
14. Add the fish cakes to the frying pan and fry on both sides until the fish cakes turn golden brown on either side and are heated in the middle.
15. Serve.

*Top Tip

Serve the fishcakes with some tartare sauce and homemade chips.

Lasagna

Ingredients

- 680g Minced Beef
- 90g Butter
- 90g Plain Flour
- 750ml Whole Milk
- 150g Mozzarella Cheese
- 10 Lasagna Sheets
- 1 Onion
- 4 Mushrooms
- 2 Red Peppers
- 1 Tablespoon of Rapeseed Oil
- 3 Cloves of Garlic
- 1 Tin of Chopped Tomatoes
- 1 Teaspoon of Oregano
- 1 Teaspoon of Basil
- Pinch of Salt
- Pinch of Ground Black Pepper

Method

1. Preheat the oven to 200°c/Gas mark 6.
2. Add 1 tablespoon of rapeseed oil to a frying pan and place over a medium/high heat.
3. Peel and chop 1 onion and 3 cloves of garlic into small pieces.
4. Add the garlic and onion pieces to the frying pan and sauté for 5 minutes, or until golden.
5. Add 680g of minced beef to the frying pan and fry for 12-15 minutes, or until all of the mince has browned.
6. Chop 2 red peppers and 4 mushrooms up and add to the frying pan. Fry for a further 6-7 minutes, until soft.

7. Pour 1 tin of chopped tomatoes into the frying pan, covering all of the ingredients.
8. Add 1 teaspoon of oregano, 1 teaspoon of basil, a pinch of salt and a pinch of ground black pepper to the ingredients and stir well.
9. Reduce the heat to low and leave to simmer.
10. Add 90g of butter to a saucepan and place over a medium heat.
11. Once the butter has melted stir in 90g of plain flour and cook for 2-3 minutes.
12. Gradually whisk in 750ml of whole milk and bring to the boil. Reduce the heat and frequently stir until the sauce starts to thicken.
13. Spoon 1/3 of the ingredients into a large greased ovenproof dish. Cover the ingredients with a layer of lasagna sheets and then pour 1/3 of the white sauce over the pasta sheets. Repeat this process two more times.
14. On the top layer sprinkle 150g of mozzarella cheese over the last layer of white sauce.
15. Place the ovenproof dish in the oven and bake for 30 minutes.
16. Serve.

*Top Tip

Serve with a side salad and some ciabatta bread.

Spaghetti Bolognese

Ingredients

- 400g Minced Beef
- 400g Tin Tomatoes, Chopped
- 400g Dried Spaghetti
- 1 Onion
- 3 Cloves of Garlic
- 1 Tablespoon of Oregano
- 1 Tablespoon of Basil
- 1 Teaspoon of Ground Black Pepper
- Salt
- 1 Tablespoon of Rapeseed Oil
- Dried Parmesan

Method

1. Add 1 tablespoon of rapeseed oil to a large saucepan and place over a medium/high heat.
2. Peel and chop 1 onion and 3 cloves of garlic up into small pieces and add to the saucepan. Add a pinch of salt to the ingredients and cook for 5-6 minutes.
3. Break up 400g of minced beef and add to the saucepan.
4. Add 1 teaspoon of ground black pepper to the mincemeat. Cook until the minced beef is brown.
5. Pour 400g of tinned chopped tomatoes into the saucepan.
6. Add 1 tablespoon of oregano and 1 tablespoon of basil to the ingredients and stir well.
7. Reduce the heat and simmer until the sauce is thick and rich, for approximately 20 minutes.
8. Fill a large saucepan with fresh cold water and add a pinch of salt.

9.   Break 400g of dried spaghetti in half and place the pasta in the saucepan of water. Place the saucepan over a medium heat and cook for 12-15 minutes, or according to the packet instructions.

10. Once the spaghetti is cooked through, drain the pasta and add to the saucepan of bolognese sauce. Mix well.

11. Sprinkle dried parmesan on top of the spaghetti bolognese.

12. Serve.

*Top Tip

Garnish the spaghetti with some fresh basil leaves. Serve the spaghetti with a side of salad and some garlic bread.

Beef Tacos

Ingredients

- 250g Minced Beef
- 20g Grated Cheddar Cheese
- 1 Clove of Garlic
- 1 Onion
- 1 Green Pepper
- 1 Red Pepper
- 4 Tablespoons of Tomato Puree
- ½ Teaspoon of Hot Paprika
- ¼ Teaspoon of Ground Cumin
- Taco Shells
- Pinch of Salt
- Pinch of Ground Black Pepper
- ½ Iceberg Lettuce
- 2 Tomatoes

Method

1. Break 250g of minced beef up and place it in a frying pan.
2. Place the frying pan over a medium heat, dry-fry the mince until it becomes brown and crumbly. Occasionally stir the mince and break any large lumps up with a spoon.
3. Chop 1 onion, 1 garlic, 1 green pepper and 1 red pepper up into small pieces. Add the ingredients to the frying pan and cook until softened.
4. Stir in ½ teaspoon of hot paprika, ¼ teaspoon of ground cumin, a pinch of salt and a pinch of ground black pepper.
5. Add 4 tablespoons of tomato puree to the ingredients and stir well.

6. Cover the frying pan and gently cook for 8-10 minutes, stirring occasionally.
7. Spoon a little of the ingredients into each of the taco shells.
8. Chop ½ iceberg lettuce up into small shredded pieces and add a little bit to each of the tacos.
9. Chop 2 tomatoes up into small pieces and place on top of the shredded iceberg lettuce.
10. Evenly sprinkle 20g of grated cheddar cheese on each of the tacos.
11. Serve.

Turkey Tacos

Ingredients

- 350g Ground Turkey
- 20g Grated Cheddar Cheese
- 3 Cloves of Garlic
- 1 Onion
- 1 Tablespoon of Rapeseed Oil
- 1 Teaspoon of Dried Oregano
- 1 Tablespoon of All Purpose Seasoning
- 1 Tablespoon Cajun Spice Mix
- ½ teaspoon of Jerk Seasoning
- Taco Shells
- ½ Iceberg Lettuce
- 2 Tomatoes
- ¼ Cucumber

Method

1. Add 1 tablespoon of rapeseed oil to a frying pan and place over a medium/high heat.
2. Peel and chop 1 onion up into small pieces and then place in the frying pan, cook for 5 minutes or until the onion has softened.
3. Peel and chop 3 cloves of garlic up into small fragments and add to the onion along with 1 teaspoon of dried oregano. Cook for 1-2 minutes.
4. Place 350g of ground turkey into the frying pan and stir.
5. Add 1 teaspoon of All-purpose seasoning, 1 teaspoon of Cajun spice mix and ½ teaspoon of Jerk seasoning to the ground turkey and mix well. Cook, for approximately 20 minutes ensuring that there are no pink bits, stirring occasionally.

6. Spoon a little of the ingredients into each of the taco shells.
7. Chop ½ iceberg lettuce into small shredded pieces and add a little bit to each of the tacos.
8. Chop 2 tomatoes and ¼ cucumber up into small pieces and place on top of the shredded iceberg lettuce.
9. Evenly sprinkle 20g of grated cheddar cheese on each of the tacos.
10. Serve.

Turkey Wraps

Ingredients
- 350g Turkey Breast
- 280g Sweetcorn, Canned
- 1 Red Chili
- ½ Lime
- 1 Tablespoon Cajun Spice Mix
- 1 Teaspoon All Purpose Seasoning
- 1 Tablespoon of Rapeseed Oil
- Tortillas
- 150ml Soured Cream
- ½ Iceberg Lettuce

Method

1. Chop 350g of turkey breast up into smaller chunks and place in a mixing bowl. Season the meat with 1 tablespoon of Cajon Spice Mix and 1 teaspoon of All-purpose seasoning.
2. Add 1 teaspoon of rapeseed oil to a frying pan and place over a medium/high heat.
3. Add the turkey chunks to the frying pan and fry for 5-6 minutes on each side, or until all of the pieces are cooked through.
4. Deseed and chop 1 red chili up into small pieces.
5. In a clean small bowl, add 280g of canned sweetcorn, the chopped red chili, and ½ lime zest and mix together to make the salsa.
6. Warm the tortillas up according to the package instructions.
7. Evenly add and spread out the turkey ingredients to each of the tortillas, along with the soured cream.

8. Chop and shred ½ iceberg lettuce and add to each of the tortillas.
9. Add a spoonful of salsa to each of the tortillas, and roll up into a wrap.
10. Serve.

Turkey Kebabs

Ingredients

- 400g Turkey Breast Fillets
- 1 Red Pepper
- 1 Green Pepper
- 1 Yellow Pepper
- 2 Large Tomatoes
- 1 Onion
- 2 Cloves of Garlic
- 1 Teaspoon of Dried Oregano
- 1 Tablespoon of Cajun Spice Mix
- 1 Tablespoon of All Purpose Seasoning
- 1 Teaspoon of Curry Powder
- ½ Teaspoon of Jerk Seasoning
- Skewers

Method

1. Dice 400g of turkey breast fillets into small chunks and place in a large mixing bowl.
2. Peel and chop 2 cloves of garlic and place in a mixing bowl.
3. Add in, 1 teaspoon of oregano, 1 tablespoon of Cajun Spice Mix, 1 tablespoon of All-purpose seasoning, 1 teaspoon of curry powder and ½ teaspoon of Jerk seasoning to the mixing bowl and blend well with the turkey chunks. For best results cover and leave to marinade in the refrigerator overnight.
4. Chop 1 red pepper, 1 green pepper, 1 yellow pepper, 2 large tomatoes and 1 onion up into small pieces, roughly 2cm long. Place the ingredients in a fresh, clean bowl and mix together.

5. Place 1 onion piece, 1 tomato piece, 1 red pepper piece, 1 yellow pepper piece, 1 green pepper piece and one chunk of turkey onto a skewer. Repeat this process in any order you like until all of the ingredients have gone.
6. Place the skewers on a baking tray and grill for 15 minutes, each side until the meat is cooked through.
7. Serve.

*Top Tip

These turkey kebabs go well with rice, pitta bread, and a homemade salad.

Turkey Meatballs

Ingredients

- 400g Turkey Mince
- 400g Tinned Chopped Tomatoes
- 400g Spaghetti
- 25g Breadcrumbs
- 3 Cloves of Garlic
- 2 Tablespoons of Rapeseed Oil
- 2 Tablespoon of Italian Seasoning
- 1 Onion
- 1 Tablespoon of Tomato Purée
- 1 Teaspoon of Oregano
- 1 Teaspoon of Basil

Method

1. Crumble 400g of turkey mince into a large mixing bowl.
2. Add 25g of breadcrumbs to the turkey mince.
3. Peel and chop 3 cloves of garlic and 1 onion up into small pieces.
4. Add half of the garlic to the mixing bowl.
5. Season the meat with 2 tablespoons of Italian seasoning, 1 teaspoon of oregano and 1 teaspoon of basil. Stir the ingredients together.
6. With your hands, shape the turkey mixture into 12 even balls, and then leave to chill for approximately 15 minutes.
7. Heat 2 tablespoons of rapeseed oil in a frying pan and place over a medium heat. Add the onion and remaining garlic to the pan and fry for five minutes, or until they have softened.
8. Place all 12 of the turkey meatballs into the frying pan and cook on a medium heat for 20-25 minutes,

until each meatball is cooked through, stirring occasionally.

9. Pour 400g of tinned chopped tomatoes into the frying pan, followed by half a tin of cold water.
10. Stir in 1 tablespoon of tomato Purée and simmer for 15 minutes, until the ingredients have thickened.
11. Serve.

*Top Tip

Serve the turkey meatballs with spaghetti, pasta or rice. Garnish with some dried parmesan and fresh basil leaves.

Linseed Chicken

Ingredients

- 400g Chicken Breast

- 150g Linseeds

- 2 Eggs

- 1 Tablespoon of Chicken Seasoning

- 1 Tablespoon of All Purpose Seasoning

- 1 Teaspoon of Ground Black Pepper

Method

1. Preheat the oven to 190c/ gas mark 5.
2. Place 400g of chicken breast in a large mixing bowl.
3. Season, the chicken with 1 tablespoon of All-purpose seasoning, 1 tablespoon of chicken seasoning and 1 teaspoon of ground black pepper.
4. Crack 2 eggs into a smaller bowl and whisk.
5. Blend 150g of linseeds and then pour out onto a large plate.
6. Dip each of the chicken breasts into the whisked egg, and then dip into the blended linseed, ensuring the linseed is evenly coated on either side of the chicken. Place the coated chicken onto a baking tray. Repeat this process until each of the chicken breasts has been coated with linseed.
7. Bake in the oven for 25-30 minutes, turning the chicken over halfway through.
8. Serve.

*Top Tip

Chop the chicken up into smaller chunks to make linseed chicken nuggets.

Turkey & Feta Cheese Burgers

Ingredients
- 450g Minced Turkey Breast
- 170g Feta Cheese
- 1 Tablespoon of Oregano
- 1 Tablespoon of All Purpose Seasoning
- 1 Teaspoon of Ground Black Pepper
- 1 egg

Method

1. Break up 450g of minced turkey breast and place it a large mixing bowl.
2. Crack and whisk 1 egg in a small bowl. Pour the whisked egg over the minced turkey.
3. Crumble 170g of feta cheese into the large mixing bowl.
4. Add 1 tablespoon of oregano, 1 tablespoon of All-purpose seasoning and 1 teaspoon of ground black pepper to the turkey and mix well.
5. Form the meat into individual, even patties, and place on a lightly oiled baking tray.
6. Grill for 10-12 minutes on each side.
7. Place the turkey & feta cheeseburgers inside some fresh bread buns and serve.

*Top Tip

You can try adding some homemade salsa, and salad to the turkey & feta cheeseburgers.

Lime Rice

Ingredients
- 250g Jasmine Rice
- 350ml Coconut Milk
- 3 Tablespoons of Desiccated Coconut
- 1 Teaspoon of Coconut Oil
- Pinch of Salt
- ½ Lime Juice
- ½ Lemon Zest

Method

1. Place 1 teaspoon of coconut oil in a saucepan and place over a medium heat.
2. Add 250g of Jasmine rice to the saucepan and cook for only 1 minute.
3. Add 3 tablespoons of desiccated coconut to the saucepan.
4. Pour in 350ml of coconut milk and stir well. Place the lid on the saucepan and bring to the boil.
5. Reduce the heat and simmer the rice for 30-35 minutes.
6. Remove from the heat and remove the lid from the saucepan.
7. Stir in ½ lime juice and ½ lime zest.
8. Add a pinch of salt.
9. Serve.

Lamb Kebabs

Ingredients
- 400g Lamb
- 1 Red Pepper
- 1 Green Pepper
- 1 Yellow Pepper
- 2 Large Tomatoes
- 1 Onion
- 2 Cloves of Garlic
- 1 Tablespoon of Mint
- 1 Tablespoon of Lamb Seasoning
- 1 Tablespoon of All Purpose Seasoning
- 1 Teaspoon of Jerk Seasoning
- 1 Teaspoon of Rosemary
- Skewers

Method

1. Dice 400g of lamb into small chunks and place in a large mixing bowl.
2. Add 2 chopped cloves of garlic, 1 teaspoon of rosemary, 1 tablespoon of lamb seasoning, 1 tablespoon of All-purpose seasoning, 1 tablespoon of mint, and 1 teaspoon of Jerk seasoning to the mixing bowl and blend well with the lamb chunks. For best results cover and leave to marinade in the refrigerator overnight.
3. Chop 1 red pepper, 1 green pepper, 1 yellow pepper, 2 large tomatoes and 1 onion up into small pieces, roughly 2cm long. Add the ingredients to a bowl and mix together.

5.   Place 1 onion piece, 1 tomato piece, 1 red pepper piece, 1 yellow pepper piece, 1 green pepper piece and one chunk of lamb onto a skewer. Repeat this process in any order you like until all of the ingredients have gone.

6.   Place the skewers on a baking tray and grill for 15 minutes on each side.

7.   Serve.

*Top Tip

These turkey kebabs go well with rice, pitta bread, and a homemade salad.

Lamb Koftas

Ingredients

- 500g Lamb Mince
- 2 Teaspoons Ground Coriander
- 3 Cloves of Garlic
- 1 Teaspoon Ground Cumin
- 1 Tablespoon Freshly Chopped Mint
- Rapeseed Oil
- Pinch of Salt
- Pinch of Ground Black Pepper

Method

1. Break up 500g of lamb mincemeat and place it in a large mixing bowl.
2. Add 2 teaspoons of ground coriander, 1 teaspoon of ground cumin, 1 tablespoon of freshly chopped mint, a pinch of salt and a pinch of ground black pepper.
3. Peel and chop 3 cloves of garlic up into small pieces and add to the mixing bowl.
4. Mix the ingredients together until they are well blended. Using your hands roll the lamb mince into eight even balls. Roll the lamb balls on a chopping board with a cupped hand to create oval shapes.
5. Thread each of the lamb ovals onto a skewer and brush with some rapeseed oil.
6. Place the koftas under the grill and cook for 8-10 minutes on each side. Alternatively, you can cook the lamb koftas on a griddle. Heat the griddle and place the koftas on top once it is hot. Cook for 4-5 minutes on each side.
7. Serve.

*Top Tip

Serve the koftas with some yogurt, salad, rice and spiced flatbread.

Cod & Broccoli Potato Pie

Ingredients
- 450g Cod Fillet
- 800g Potatoes
- 120g Broccoli Florets, Cooked
- 120g Leeks
- 100g Butter
- 50g Flour
- 1 Pint of Milk
- 1 Onion
- 2 Teaspoons Fresh Parsley, Chopped

Method

1. Preheat the oven to 180c/ gas mark 4.
2. Poach 450g of cod in a pint of milk until the fish is cooked. Flake the cod and leave to one side, keep the milk for your sauce.
3. Chop 1 onion and 120g of leeks up into small pieces.
4. Place a frying pan over a medium/high heat and add a little bit of butter to the pan.
5. Add the onion and leeks to the frying pan and fry until they become transparent.
6. Add in 50g of flour to the frying pan. Constantly stir the ingredients and cook for a further 4-5 minutes until a roux is formed.
7. Gradually pour in the milk while still stirring the roux.
8. Add the flaked cod and 120g of cooked broccoli florets to the pan and simmer for 5 minutes.
9. Pour the fish mixture into a large ovenproof dish and set aside.
10. Peel and chop 800g of potatoes. Place the potatoes pieces in a large saucepan and boil until tender. Drain

the potatoes and add in some butter. Mash the potatoes until they become soft and creamy.

11. Spread the mash potatoes over the top of the fish mixture.

12. Place the ovenproof dish in the oven and cook for 20-25 minutes. Place the fish pie under the grill before removing it from the oven for a few minutes to brown the potato.

13. Serve.

*Top Tip

Try serving this cod & broccoli potato pie with some vegetables.

Lamb Burgers

Ingredients

- 450g Lean Lamb Mince
- ½ Onion
- 4 Teaspoons of Rosemary
- 2 Cloves of Garlic, chopped
- 1 Teaspoon Mint
- 2 Teaspoons of Rapeseed Oil
- 1 Teaspoon Lamb Seasoning
- 2 Teaspoons Oats
- 1 Tablespoon of Water

Method

1. Preheat the oven to 190c/ gas mark 5.
2. Place 450g of lean lamb mince in a large mixing bowl.
3. Grate ½ onion into the mixing bowl.
4. Add 4 teaspoons of rosemary, 1 teaspoon of mint, 1 teaspoon of lamb seasoning, 2 teaspoons of oats, 1 tablespoon of water and 2 cloves of chopped garlic to the lamb mincemeat.
5. Mix all of the ingredients together and form into even sized burgers.
6. Place the lamb burgers on a baking tray and lightly flatten each one with the palm of your hand.
7. Brush each of the burgers with rapeseed oil.
8. Place the baking tray in the oven and cook for 20 minutes, turning the burgers halfway through.

*Top Tip

You can make the lamb burgers as thick or as thin as you like. You can also add more or less seasoning to suit your taste.

Shepherd's Pie

Ingredients

- 900g Potatoes
- 500g Mince Meat
- 500ml Beef Stock
- 85g Butter
- 1 Onion
- 2-3 Carrots
- 10ml Milk
- 1 Tablespoon Rapeseed Oil
- 1 Tablespoon Butter
- 2 Tablespoons Tomato Purée
- 1 Teaspoon Worcestershire Sauce

Method

1. Preheat the oven to 180c/ gas mark 4.
2. Peel and chop 1 onion and 2-3 carrots.
3. Add 1 tablespoon of rapeseed oil to a large frying pan or wok and place over a medium heat. Add in the onion and carrots and cook for a few minutes until they have softened. Once the vegetables have softened increase the heat to high.
4. Crumble in 500g of mince meat and cook until it has browned. Drain out any excess fat.
5. Add in 2 tablespoons of tomato Purée and 1 teaspoon of Worcestershire sauce. Fry for a few minutes.
6. Pour in 500ml of beef stock and bring to a simmer.
7. Cover the pan and cook for a further 30-40 minutes. Uncover halfway through and give the ingredients a quick stir.
8. Peel and chop 900g of potatoes. Place the potatoes in a large saucepan and cover them with fresh cold

water. Place the saucepan over a medium/high heat and boil until the potatoes have softened.

9. Once the potatoes are soft drain any excess water and then add in 10ml of milk and a tablespoon of butter. Mash the ingredients together.

10. Pour the mincemeat out evenly into a large ovenproof dish.

11. Cover the mincemeat with the mash potatoes. Ruffle the mashed potato with a fork.

12. Place the ovenproof dish in the oven and bake for 20-25 minutes.

13. Remove from the oven.

14. Serve.

*Top Tip

You can freeze the shepherd's pie before placing it in the oven for up to 1 month. To cook from frozen cook at 160c/gas mark 3 for at least 1 hour, until the center is piping hot and cooked through. Serve the Shepherd's pie with gravy and vegetables.

Bubble & Squeak

Ingredients

- 450g Cooked Mashed Potatoes
- 225g Cooked Cabbage
- 200g Grated Cheddar Cheese
- 1 Onion
- 25g Butter
- 1 Tablespoon Plain Flour
- 1 Tablespoon Rapeseed Oil
- Pinch of Salt
- Pinch of Ground Black Pepper

Method

1. Peel and chop 1 onion into small pieces.
2. Add 25g of butter to a large frying pan and place over a medium heat until all of the butter has melted.
3. Add the onion to the frying pan and cook for 10 minutes until soft.
4. Empty the soft onion into a large mixing bowl.
5. Add 450g of cooked mashed potato to the onion and 225g of cooked shredded cabbage.
6. Season the vegetables with a pinch of salt and a pinch of ground black pepper.
7. Mix the ingredients together well.
8. Lightly flour your hands and then shape the vegetable mixture into four rough cakes, approximately 2cm thick.
9. In a clean frying pan add 1 tablespoon of rapeseed oil and place over a medium heat.
10. Place the vegetable cakes in the pan and fry for 15 minutes, turn once half way through. Fry until crisp and golden brown.

11. Remove the bubble and squeak from the frying pan and place on a plate.
12. Sprinkle the grated cheese over the bubble and squeak while it is still hot so that it melts in.
13. Serve.

*Top Tip

Try serving the bubble and squeak with some sausages.

Sweet & Sour Pork

Ingredients
- 500g Pork, Diced
- 350g Rice
- 125g Sweet Corn
- 100g Bean Sprouts
- 2 Carrots
- 1 Onion
- 1 Red Pepper
- 2 Spring Onions
- 2 Tablespoons Rice Wine
- 1 Teaspoon Ground Ginger
- 1 Tin of Pineapple Chunks
- 1 Clove of Garlic
- 1 Tablespoon Demerara Sugar
- 2 Tablespoons Tomato Ketchup
- 2 Tablespoons Soya Sauce
- 2 Tablespoons Rapeseed Oil

Method

1. Preheat the oven to 180c/ gas mark 4.
2. Add 2 tablespoons of rapeseed oil to a large frying pan and place over a medium/high heat.
3. Add 500g of diced pork to the frying pan and brown.
4. Peel and chop 1 onion, 1 clove of garlic and 2 carrots. Add the vegetables to the frying pan and soften for 5 minutes.
5. Peel and chop 1 red pepper and then add it to the pan.
6. Pour in the juice from 1 tin of pineapple chunks into a mixing bowl. Add in 1 teaspoon of ground

ginger, 2 tablespoons of rice wine, 1 teaspoon of demerara sugar, 2 tablespoons of tomato ketchup and 2 tablespoons of soya sauce. Mix the ingredients together well.

7. Pour the liquid over the pork and vegetables and bring to a boil.

8. Remove the frying pan from the heat and pour the ingredients into an ovenproof dish. Cover the dish with a lid and cook in the oven for 40-45 minutes.

9. Cook 350g of rice according to the instructions on the packet.

10. Add 2 spring onions, 100g of bean sprouts and 125g of sweet corn to the pork.

11. Serve the sweet and sour pork on a bed of rice.

*Top Tip

You can also add a side of vegetables to this sweet and sour pork dish.

Sausage & Bean Hotpot

Ingredients
- 8 Thick Pork Sausages
- 800g Baked Beans
- 400g Tinned Cannellini Beans
- 400g Tinned Chopped Tomatoes
- 125ml Water
- 30ml Tomato Purée
- 2 Tablespoons Rapeseed Oil
- 2 Red Peppers
- 1 Onion
- 1 Teaspoon Rosemary
- 1 Teaspoon Parsley
- ½ Teaspoon Chili Flakes
- Pinch of Ground Black Pepper

Method

1. Preheat the oven to 180c/gas mark 4.
2. Cut 8 thick sausages in half, lengthways.
3. Add 2 tablespoons of rapeseed oil to a large frying pan and place over a medium/high heat.
4. Add the sausages to the frying pan and brown.
5. Chop 1 onion and 2 red pepper into small pieces. Add the onion and pepper to the frying pan and sauté for 3-4 minutes.
6. Add 1 teaspoon of rosemary, 1 teaspoon of parsley and ½ teaspoon of chili flakes into the ingredients.
7. Pour in 800g of baked beans, 400g of tinned cannellini beans and 400g of tinned chopped tomatoes and stir well.
8. Add 30ml of tomato Purée and a pinch of ground black pepper to the ingredients and bring to the boil.

9. Pour the hot pot out into an oven proof dish and place in the oven for 20-25 minutes. Stir the hot pot once, half way through the cooking time.
10. Serve.

*Top Tip

You can cut the sausages up into smaller pieces if you prefer. This sausage and bean hotpot tastes nice with some crusty French stick.

Beef & Onion Pie

Ingredients

- 400g Beef, Diced
- 3 Carrots
- 2 Onions
- 2 Tablespoons Plain Flour
- 2 Tablespoons Mixed Herbs
- 1 Large Sheet Ready Rolled Flaky Pastry
- 1 Egg
- 1 Vegetable Stock Cube
- 1 Teaspoon Rapeseed Oil

Method

1. Preheat the oven to 190c/gas mark 5.
2. Add 1 teaspoon of rapeseed oil to a frying pan and place over a medium heat.
3. Add 400g of diced beef to the frying pan and brown.
4. Peel and chop 3 carrots and 2 onions and then add the vegetables to the frying pan. Stir for 5 minutes.
5. Add 2 tablespoons of mixed herbs to the frying pan and cook for a few more minutes.
6. Add 1 vegetable stock cube to a measuring jug and add some boiling water to make the stock.
7. Add 2 tablespoons of plain flour to the beef and cook for a further 2-3 minutes.
8. Gradually add in the vegetable stock to the frying pan, constantly stirring the ingredients to prevent any lumps from forming. Add enough vegetable stock in to make a thick gravy.
9. Reduce the heat and cover with a lid. Simmer the ingredients for 45 minutes, until the beef is tender.

10. Once the meat is tender remove the frying pan from the heat. Pour the ingredients out into an ovenproof dish and allow to cool.
11. Line, the top rim of the oven proof dish with a thin strip of the ready, rolled flaky pastry sheet.
12. Crack and beat 1 egg in a small bowl. Brush the top of the pastry with the beaten egg.
13. Cover the pie filling with the remaining pastry. Gently press the pastry edges down with a fork into the pastry strip lining the rim of the oven proof dish.
14. Make a slit in the top of the pastry with a knife. This is to allow the steam to escape from the pie while cooking.
15. Brush the pastry with the remaining egg.
16. Place the ovenproof dish in the oven and cook for 25-30 minutes.
17. Serve.

*Top Tip

This beef and onion pie tastes delicious when served with some mashed potatoes and vegetables.

Braised Lamb

Ingredients
- 8 Lamb Shanks
- 500ml Lamb Stock
- 350ml White Wine
- 300ml Beef Stock
- 25g Plain Flour
- 1 Onion
- 4 Garlic Cloves
- 2 Carrots
- A Few Sprigs of Fresh Rosemary
- 3 Bay Leafs
- 2 Tablespoons Plain Flour
- 2 Tablespoons Rapeseed Oil
- 1 Tablespoon Tomato Purée

Method

1. Preheat the oven to 190c/gas mark 5.
2. Coat 8 lamb shanks with 2 tablespoons of plain flour.
3. Add 2 tablespoons of rapeseed oil to a frying pan and place over a medium/high heat.
4. Place the lamb shanks into the frying pan and brown for 7-10 minutes.
5. Peel and chop 2 carrots, 4 cloves of garlic and 1 onion. Add the vegetables to the pan and soften for 5 minutes.
6. Add in a few sprigs of fresh rosemary and 3 bay leafs and cook for a few more minutes.
7. Stir in 1 Tablespoon of tomato purée.
8. Pour over 350ml of white wine and 300ml of beef stock.

9. Cover the pan with a lid and bring to a simmer for 1½-2 hours until the lamb is tender.
10. Remove the lamb shanks from the sauce and set aside.
11. Place the sauce back over a medium heat and boil it down for approximately 15 minutes, until the sauce is rich and glossy.
12. Place the lamb shanks back in the sauce and cook for a few more minutes before serving.
13. Serve.

*Top Tip

If you need to add a few tablespoons of water to the sauce, then you can do so before adding the lamb shanks back into the pan. Braised lamb tastes delicious with roast potatoes and vegetables.

Vegetable Lasagna

Ingredients

- 320g Chopped Tomatoes, Tinned
- 200g Lasagna Sheets
- 300ml Water
- 900ml Water
- 100g Red Lentils
- 90g Cheddar Cheese
- 90g Dried Skimmed Milk Powder
- 90g Plain Flour
- 2 Onions
- 2 Carrots
- 80g Mushrooms
- 2 Red Peppers
- 2 Aubergines
- 2 Cloves of Garlic
- 1 Green Pepper
- 1 courgette
- 8 Tablespoons Rapeseed Oil
- 1 Tablespoon Tomato Puree
- 1 Teaspoon Mixed Herbs
- Pinch of Ground Black Pepper

Method

1. Preheat the oven to 180c/gas mark 4.
2. Place 100g of red lentils in a medium sized saucepan and cover with water. Place the saucepan over a medium/high heat and bring to the boil. Then simmer for 15-20 minutes.
3. Peel and chop 2 onions, 2 carrots, 2 red peppers, 1 green pepper and 2 cloves of garlic. Place the

vegetables in a large saucepan and pour in a little bit of water.

4. Chop up 80g of mushrooms, 1 courgette, and 2 aubergines and add them to the vegetables.

5. Place the saucepan over a high heat and cook until the vegetables turn soft.

6. Add in the lentils, 1 teaspoon of mixed herbs and 1 tablespoon of tomato puree.

7. Pour in 320g of tinned chopped tomatoes and 900ml of water and stir the ingredients together. Bring to the boil.

8. Make up the dried skimmed milk powder according to the instructions.

9. In a separate saucepan add 90g of plain flour and a little bit of the water. Pour the mixture into the milk.

10. Place the saucepan over a medium heat and bring to the boil, constantly stirring the ingredients.

11. Add in 90g of cheddar cheese and stir.

12. Layer a large oven proof dish with the vegetable sauce, then add a layer of lasagna sheets, followed by a layer of cheese sauce. Repeat this process one more time.

13. Place the ovenproof dish in the oven and bake for 50-60 minutes.

14. Serve.

*Top Tip

You can substitute the cheddar cheese for a cheese of your choice such of mozzarella. This vegetable lasagna tastes delicious when served with a side of salad and some freshly made garlic bread.

Bean Burgers

Ingredients
- 2x 400g Canned Mixed Beans, Drained
- 100g Dried Breadcrumbs
- 3 Cloves of Garlic
- 1 Egg
- 1 Tablespoon of Chili Powder
- 1 Tablespoon Cumin
- ½ Green Pepper
- ½ Onion

Method

1. Preheat the oven to 190c/gas mark 5. Lightly oil a baking tray.
2. Pour the mixed beans into a large mixing bowl and mash until they become thick and pasty. Alternatively, you can puree the beans in a blender.
3. Place ½ green pepper, ½ onion, 3 cloves of garlic in a blender and blend for 30-50 seconds. Stir the ingredients into the mashed beans.
4. Crack 1 egg into a small bowl and whisk.
5. Add 1 tablespoon of chili powder and 1 tablespoon of cumin to the egg and lightly whisk.
6. Stir the egg mixture into the beans.
7. Add in 100g of dried breadcrumbs to the mixing bowl and blend until the mixture becomes sticky and holds together. If the mixture is too wet add some more breadcrumbs.
8. Divide the mixture up into even burgers.
9. Place the bean burgers on top of the lightly oiled baking tray and place in the oven. Cook for 10-12 minutes or until the burgers are golden brown,

carefully turn the bean burgers over and repeat on the other side.

10. Serve.

*Top Tip

Serve the bean burgers in some fresh soft bread rolls with a little bit of salad and a side of salsa and homemade potato wedges.

Creamy Chicken & Broccoli Pie

Ingredients
- 5 Chicken Thighs, Skinless & Boneless
- 1 Broccoli
- 2 Onions
- 2 Cloves of Garlic
- 1 Bay Leaf
- A Handful of Fresh Parsley
- 2 Tablespoons Plain Flour
- 1 Pint Chicken Stock
- 1 Packet of Ready Rolled Puff Pastry
- 75ml Double Cream
- 1 Egg
- 1 Tablespoon Rapeseed Oil
- Salt
- Ground Black Pepper

Method

1. Preheat the oven to 200c/gas mark 6.
2. Cut the skinless and boneless chicken thighs up into large chunks of meat.
3. Chop 1 broccoli up into florets and place in a medium sized saucepan. Cover the broccoli with water and place over a high heat. Blanch the broccoli and then remove from the heat and drain.
4. Add 1 tablespoon of rapeseed oil to a large saucepan and place over a high heat.
5. Add the chicken chunks to the saucepan along with 1 bay leaf.
6. Season the chicken to taste with some salt and ground black pepper.

7. Brown the chicken for at least 5-6 minutes, ensuring that you stir throughout until all of the chicken chunks have browned.

8. Peel and chop 2 onions and 2 cloves of garlic. Place the vegetables in the large saucepan and cook for a further 1-2 minutes.

9. Sprinkle in 2 tablespoons of plain flour. Cook for 1-2 minutes before adding 1/3 of the chicken stock. Constantly stir the ingredients together to avoid any lumps from forming. Once the sauce has thickened gradually pour in the remaining chicken stock and 75ml of double cream.

10. Reduce the heat to low and cook the chicken uncovered for 15-20 minutes to allow the sauce to thicken as the chicken cooks.

11. Stir in the blanched broccoli florets.

12. Add in a handful of fresh parsley.

13. Remove the saucepan from the heat and pour the ingredients out into an ovenproof dish.

14. Roughly cut 1 packet of ready rolled puff pastry to the same size as the top of the ovenproof dish. Place the pastry over the top of the chicken mixture.

15. Score the top of the pastry with a knife and make a small hole, this is to ensure that the steam can escape from the pie.

16. Crack and beat 1 egg in a small bowl.

17. Brush the pastry with the beaten egg.

18. Place the ovenproof dish in the oven and cook for 35-40 minutes, or until the pie is golden brown and cooked through.

19. Serve.

*Top Tip

This chicken and broccoli pie tastes delicious when served with some green vegetables and mashed potatoes.

Stuffed Jacket Potato

Ingredients

- 2 Large Potatoes
- 2 Slices of Bacon
- 2 Spring Onions
- 150g Cottage Cheese
- 20g Cheddar Cheese, Grated
- 2 Tablespoons Chives
- 1 Egg Yolk
- 2 Tablespoon Virgin Olive Oil
- Pinch of Salt
- Pinch of Ground Black Pepper

Method

1. Preheat the oven to 200c/ gas mark 6.
2. Wash 2 large potatoes and then rub the skins all over with some of the olive oil and salt.
3. Lightly stab the potatoes a couple of times with a sharp knife. Rap each of the potatoes up in a layer of tin foil and then place on a baking tray. Place the baking tray in the oven and cook for 1 hour, or until the potatoes have softened and cooked through.
4. Cut 2 slices of bacon up into small pieces.
5. Heat a frying pan and dry fry the bacon pieces until they turn crispy.
6. Finely chop 2 spring onions up and add them to the bacon. Cook for a further 2 minutes before removing the frying pan from the heat and setting aside.
7. Remove the foil from the potatoes and cut each one in half.
8. Scoop the middles of the potatoes out and place them in a large mixing bowl. Leave enough potato in the skins to ensure that the potatoes keep their shape.

9. Mash the middles of the potatoes up with a masher.
10. Add in the bacon and spring onions to the potato middles.
11. Pour in 150g of cottage cheese and 1 egg yolk.
12. Add in 2 tablespoons of chives and a pinch of salt and ground black pepper.
13. Mix the ingredients together well.
14. Spoon the potato mixture back into the skins of the potatoes.
15. Sprinkle the tops of each potato with some grated cheddar cheese and then lightly drizzle with some virgin olive oil.
16. Place the potatoes back on the baking tray and in the oven. Cook for a further 5-10 minutes or until the cheese has started to melt and turned golden.
17. Serve.

*Top Tip

You can season your potatoes to taste. You can also experiment with the stuffing ingredients to suit your tastes such as by adding red or green peppers. These stuffed jacket potatoes taste wonderful with a side of fresh salad.

Toad in the Hole

Ingredients
- 8 Pork Sausages
- 225g Plain Flour
- 250ml Milk
- 4 Eggs
- 1 Tablespoon Rapeseed Oil
- Pinch of Salt
- Pinch of Ground Pepper

Method

1. Preheat the oven to 200c/ gas mark 6.
2. Add 1 tablespoon of rapeseed oil to the bottom of a deep baking tray.
3. Add 8 pork sausages to the baking tray, making sure that you spread them out in a single layer. Place the baking tray in the oven and cook for 10 minutes.
4. Place 225g of plain flour in a large mixing bowl and add 4 eggs and 125ml of the milk. Whisk the ingredients together until it becomes smooth. Gradually whisk in the other half of the milk and add in a pinch of salt and a pinch of ground black pepper. Keep whisking until the batter is smooth and free of lumps.
5. Take the baking tray out of the oven and pour in the batter, ensuring that all of the sausages are ¾ covered.
6. Place the baking tray back inside of the oven and bake for 35-40 minutes, or until the Yorkshire pudding has risen and browned in the center.
7. Serve hot.

*Top Tip

You can try adding different flavored sausages to create a different flavored toad in the hole. You can also add herbs to the Yorkshire pudding such as sage.

Tuna Steaks

Ingredients
- 2 Tuna Steaks
- 2 Tablespoons Rapeseed Oil
- ¼ Cucumber
- 1 Spring Onion
- 1 Tomato
- ¼ Red Chili
- 1 Tablespoon Olive Oil
- 1 Tablespoon Chopped Parsley
- ½ Tablespoon Lemon Juice
- Salt
- Ground Black Pepper
- Pinch of Coriander

Method

1. Pour 2 tablespoons of rapeseed oil into a food bag and then add 2 tuna steaks and rub together. Leave the tuna steaks for 30 minutes.
2. Chop ¼ of a cucumber, 1 tomato, 1 spring onion and ¼ of a red chili up into finely diced pieces and place in a small mixing bowl.
3. Add in 1 tablespoon of olive oil, 1 tablespoon of chopped parsley and ½ a tablespoon of lemon juice to the small mixing bowl. Season with a pinch of salt and a pinch of ground black pepper. Stir the ingredients together.
4. Add 1 pinch of salt, 1 pinch of black pepper and a pinch of coriander to a mortar and pestle and mash the ingredients together. Pour the seasoning onto a plate or a chopping board.

5. Take out the tuna steaks and place them on top of the seasoning, ensuring both sides of the tuna steaks have salt, pepper, and coriander on them.

6. Heat a griddle or a frying pan over a medium/high heat. Add the tuna steaks to the pan and cook for 2 minutes either side. You may need a little longer depending on the thickness of the tuna steaks.

7. Remove the steaks from the heat and place on a plate.

8. Allow the tuna steaks to cool for a couple of minutes before spooning on the fresh relish.

9. Serve.

*Top Tip

Meaty fish is best served slightly pink in the middle.

Macaroni Cheese

Ingredients

- 250g Macaroni Pasta
- 250g Cheddar Cheese, Grated
- 50g Butter
- 50g Plain Flour
- 600ml Milk
- 60g Parmesan Cheese, Grated
- 1 Teaspoon of Nutmeg
- 1 Teaspoon of Cinnamon

Method

1. Place 250g of macaroni pasta in a large saucepan full of boiling water and place over a medium heat. Cook for 6-8 minutes before draining well and setting aside.
2. Preheat the grill to hot.
3. Add 50g of butter in a large saucepan and place over a low/medium heat.
4. Add in 50g of plain flour to the butter and stir together to form a roux.
5. Gradually whisk in 600ml of milk. Constantly stir the mixture until a thick and smooth sauce is created.
6. Add 1 teaspoon of nutmeg and 1 teaspoon of cinnamon to the sauce and stir well.
7. Remove the saucepan from the heat.
8. Add half of the cheddar cheese to the sauce and stir until all of the cheese has melted.
9. Pour in the macaroni and stir the ingredients together.
10. Pour the macaroni cheese out into an ovenproof dish.
11. Sprinkle the macaroni with the remaining cheddar cheese.

12. Add 60g of parmesan cheese to the top of the macaroni cheese.
13. Place the ovenproof dish under the grill and cook until the cheese has browned, for approximately 15-18 minutes.
14. Serve.

Cauliflower Cheese

Ingredients
- 1 Large Cauliflower
- 500ml Milk
- 120g Cheddar Cheese
- 50g Butter
- 5 Tablespoons of Plain Flour

Method

1. Fill a large saucepan up with fresh cold water and place over a medium-high heat. Bring the water to a boil.
2. Preheat the oven to 220c/ gas mark 7.
3. Break 1 large cauliflower up into smaller pieces and remove the leaves.
4. Add the cauliflower pieces to the saucepan of boiling water and cook for 5-7 minutes.
5. Drain the cauliflower and then pour it out into an ovenproof dish.
6. Pour 500ml of milk into a clean saucepan and place over a low-medium heat.
7. Whisk in 50g of milk and 5 tablespoons of plain flour. Whisk the ingredients together until all of the butter has melted and the sauce has thickened.
8. Remove the saucepan from the heat and stir in 100g of cheddar cheese.
9. Pour the cheese sauce into the ovenproof dish, covering all of the cauliflower.
10. Sprinkle 20g of cheddar cheese over the top of the cauliflower.
11. Place the ovenproof dish in the oven and bake for 20 minutes.

12. Serve.

*Top Tip

Cauliflower cheese is a perfect side for poultry dishes.

Salmon & Scrambled Eggs on Toast

Ingredients

- 60g Smoked Salmon Trimmings4l
- 25g Butter
- 3 Eggs
- 2 Slices of Whole Wheat Bread
- 1 Tablespoon of Fresh Chopped Chives
- Pinch of Ground Black Pepper

Method

1. Crack and beat 3 eggs in a medium sized mixing bowl.
2. Add in 1 tablespoon of freshly chopped chives to the mixing bowl and a pinch of ground black pepper.
3. Add 25g of butter to a frying pan and place over a low/medium heat.
4. Pour the eggs into the frying pan and gently cook, occasionally stirring until they have softly scrambled for approximately 4-5 minutes.
5. Toast 2 slices of whole wheat bread and lightly butter.
6. Remove the eggs from heat and fold in 60g of smoked salmon trimmings.
7. Spoon the eggs and salmon on top of the toasted bread.
8. Serve.

*Top Tip

You can add more salmon to suit your personal preference. Season to taste.

Creamy Pollok & Vegetable Pasta Bake

Ingredients

- 300g Pasta Bows
- 250g Skinless and Boneless Pollok
- 600ml Milk
- 40g Butter
- 40g Plain Flour
- 400g Frozen Mixed Vegetables
- 100g Mild Cheddar Cheese, Grated
- 1 Teaspoon Mustard

Method

1. Preheat the oven to 220c/ gas mark 7.
2. Gently poach 250g of skinless and boneless Pollok in a little milk.
3. Pour 300g of pasta bows into a large saucepan of fresh water and place over a medium/high heat. Cook for approximately 12-15 minutes, or according to the instructions on the packet.
4. Add 40g of butter to a large saucepan and place over a medium heat.
5. Stir in 40g of plain flour and cook for 1-2 minutes.
6. Gradually whisk in the rest of the milk until the sauce becomes creamy.
7. Add 400g of frozen mixed vegetables to the sauce and gently simmer for 5-6 minutes.
8. Remove the saucepan from the heat.
9. Flake in the Pollock and stir.
10. Add 1 teaspoon of mustard and 2/3 of the cheddar cheese to the sauce and mix the ingredients together.
11. Stir in the pasta bows and mix well.
12. Evenly pour the ingredients out into an ovenproof dish.

13. Sprinkle the rest of the cheddar cheese on top of the pasta bake.
14. Place the ovenproof dish in the oven and bake for 10-12 minutes.
15. Serve.

*Top Tip

You can substitute the Pollock with other white fish such as cod, coley, or hake.

Pasta Prima Vera

Ingredients

- 350g Pasta Bows
- 1 Tin of Chopped Tomatoes
- 4 Tablespoons of Cream Cheese
- 60g Grated Cheddar Cheese
- 85g Frozen Peas
- 2 Courgettes
- 1 Carrot
- 1 Head of Broccoli

Method

1. Pour 350g of pasta bows into a large saucepan full of fresh water and place over a medium/high heat.
2. Chop 2 courgettes up into small pieces and add to the pasta.
3. Break up 1 head of broccoli up into small florets and place in the saucepan.
4. Peel and chop 1 carrot up into small thin pieces and add to the pasta.
5. Cook for approximately 12-15 minutes or according to the instructions on the packet.
6. Add 85g of frozen peas to the ingredients 3-4 minutes before you remove the saucepan from the heat.
7. Drain the pasta and the vegetables in a colander.
8. Pour 1 tin of chopped tomatoes into a large saucepan and place over a medium heat.
9. Add 4 tablespoons of cream cheese to the tomatoes and stir until all of the cream cheese has melted.

10. Pour in the pasta and vegetables and stir well.
11. Remove the saucepan from the heat.
12. Divide the ingredients up and serve in a bowl or on a plate.
13. Sprinkle the grated cheese on top of each of the pasta dishes and serve.

Desserts

Apple & Mango Crumble

Ingredients
- 450g Apples
- 175g Plain Flour/ All Purpose Flour
- 115g Caster Sugar
- 115g Cold Butter
- 1 Mango

Method

1. Preheat the oven to 180c/ gas mark 5.
2. Peel 450g of apples and 1 whole mango, discard any skin, stones, and pips. Chop the mango and apples up into chunky pieces and place in a large saucepan.
3. Fill the saucepan up with fresh cold water and place on a medium/high heat. Boil the fruit for approximately 15 minutes.
4. Pour 115g of sugar into a large mixing bowl. Add in 175g of plain flour/ all-purpose flour, and mix together.
5. Add 115g of cold butter to the mixing bowl and blend the ingredients together with your hands.
6. Drain the mango and apples from the saucepan and evenly pour the fruit out into an ovenproof dish.
7. Add a generous layer of crumble topping to the top of the fruit.
8. Place the ovenproof dish in the oven and bake until the top of the crumble turns golden brown, for approximately 30 minutes.
9. Serve.

*Top Tip

Serve this apple & mango fruit crumble with some custard or vanilla ice cream.

Banana Cake

Ingredients
- 190g Self Raising Flour
- 150g Caster Sugar
- 60ml Whole Milk
- 25g Butter
- 2 Ripe Bananas
- 2 Teaspoon Vanilla Extract
- 1 Egg

Method

1. Preheat the oven to 170c/ gas mark 3.
2. Line and generously grease a loaf tin with some butter.
3. Place 25g of butter in a small saucepan and place over a medium heat, until all of the butter has melted.
4. Add in 150g of caster sugar to the saucepan, along with 2 teaspoons of vanilla extract and stir well.
5. Remove the saucepan from the heat and pour the ingredients into a large mixing bowl.
6. Mash 2 ripe bananas up and add them to the mixing bowl. Blend the ingredients together.
7. Crack 1 egg into a small bowl and beat well. Add the egg to the banana mixture.
8. Add 190g of self-raising flour to the mixing bowl and stir well before pouring in 60ml of whole milk.
9. Pour the ingredients out into the greased loaf tin and bake in the oven for 30-35 minutes.
10. Serve hold or cold.

*Top Tip

Sprinkle the top of the banana cake with demerara sugar before placing inside of the oven to create a crunchier topping.

Carrot Muffins

Ingredients
- 250g Carrots
- 150g Butter
- 200g Caster Sugar
- 200g Self Raising Flour
- 2 Teaspoons of Cinnamon
- 2 Teaspoons of Baking Powder
- 2 Eggs
- 135g Sultanas
- 60g Nuts
- 1 Orange, Zest

Method

1. Preheat the oven to 200c/ gas mark 6 and line a muffin tray with 12 muffin cases.
2. Add 150g of butter to a saucepan and place over a medium heat, until the all of the butter has melted. Remove the saucepan from the heat.
3. Peel 250g of carrots, discard the skin. Grate the carrots into a large mixing bowl.
4. Add 200g of caster sugar and 150g of melted butter to the mixing bowl and stir together.
5. Sift in 200g of self-raising flour and add 2 teaspoons of cinnamon and 2 teaspoons of baking power.
6. Crack and beat 2 eggs in a small bowl. Pour the eggs into the mixing bowl and blend together.
7. Add 135g of Sultanas, 60g of nuts and the zest from one orange to the ingredients and stir well.

8. Divide the muffin mixture equally between the 12 muffin cases.
9. Place the muffin tray in the oven and bake for 20-25 minutes.
10. Serve warm or cold.

Chocolate Coconut Flapjack

Ingredients
- 250g Rolled Oats
- 4 Tablespoons of Golden Syrup
- 100g Brown Sugar
- 125g Butter
- 85g Desiccated Coconut
- 125g Milk Chocolate

Method

1. Preheat the oven to 180c/ gas mark 4. Lightly grease a square baking tin approximately 20cm.
2. Add 125g of butter to a large saucepan and place over a medium heat, until all of the butter has melted.
3. Add 4 tablespoons of golden syrup and 100g of brown sugar to the saucepan and occasionally stir until all of the ingredients have melted.
4. Stir in 250g of rolled oats and 85g of desiccated coconut. Stir the ingredients together until all of the oats are coated.
5. Remove the saucepan from the heat and pour the ingredients out into the baking tin.
6. Place the baking tin into the oven and bake for 30-40 minutes.
7. Break 125g of milk chocolate up into little pieces and place inside of a glass heat-proof bowl. Add the bowl to a pan of water and place over a low-medium heat to melt the chocolate. Stir the chocolate frequently until it has all melted. Remove the pan from the heat.

8. Evenly pour out and spread the melted chocolate on top of the cooked flapjack. Place the flapjack in the refrigerator to set.
9. Serve warm or cold.

Coconut Rocks

Ingredients
- 200g Self Raising Flour
- 100g Butter
- 75g Caster Sugar
- 1 Medium Egg
- 100g Desiccated Coconut

Method

1. Preheat the oven to 180c/ gas mark 6 and lightly grease a baking tray.
2. Sieve 200g of self-raising flour into a large mixing bowl.
3. Rub 100g of butter into the flour, using your fingertips until the mixture begins to look like breadcrumbs.
4. Add 75g of caster sugar and 100g of desiccated coconut into the mixing bowl and mix together.
5. Crack and beat 1 egg into a small bowl. Pour the egg into the mixing bowl and blend the ingredients together.
6. Divide the mixture up into 12 even rocky heaps and place on the baking tray.
7. Bake in the oven for 12-15 minutes or until they are golden brown and firm to touch.
8. Leave to cool before serving.

Cranberry Flapjacks

Ingredients
- 250g Rolled Oats
- 4 Tablespoons of Golden Syrup
- 100g Brown Sugar
- 125g Butter
- 125g Cranberries

Method

1. Preheat the oven to 180c/ gas mark 4. Lightly grease a square baking tin approximately 20cm.
2. Add 125g of butter to a large saucepan and place over a medium heat, until all of the butter has melted.
3. Add 4 tablespoons of golden syrup and 100g of brown sugar to the saucepan and occasionally stir until all of the ingredients have melted.
4. Stir in 250g of rolled oats and 125g of cranberries. Stir the ingredients together until all of the oats are coated.
5. Remove the saucepan from the heat and pour the ingredients out into the baking tin.
6. Place the baking tin in the oven and bake for 30-40 minutes.
7. Serve warm or cold.

Peanut Butter Cookies

Ingredients

- 200g Peanut Butter
- 175g Caster Sugar
- 1 Egg

Method

1. Preheat the oven to 180c/ gas mark 4 and line two baking trays with baking paper.
2. Place 200g of peanut butter, soft or crunchy in a large mixing bowl.
3. Add 175g of caster sugar to the peanut butter and mix together.
4. Add 1 egg to the mixing bowl and blend together until the ingredients form a dough.
5. Divide the mixture into small chunks of dough, roughly the size of a cherry tomato. Place the chunks of dough onto the baking trays, ensuring that they are spaced well apart.
6. Using a fork, press down on each of the dough chunks to squash them down a little bit.
7. Place the baking trays in the oven and bake for 12-15 minutes or until the cookies are golden around the edges.
8. Leave to cool and serve.

*Top Tip

Once you have formed your cookies, you can freeze them for up to two months and cook them straight from frozen.

Raspberry Crumble

Ingredients
- 350g Raspberries
- 175g Plain Flour/ All Purpose Flour
- 115g Caster Sugar
- 115g Cold Butter

Method

1. Preheat the oven to 180c/ gas mark 5.
2. Place 350g of raspberries in a baking dish and sprinkle with a generous teaspoon of sugar.
3. Pour 115g of sugar into a large mixing bowl. Add in 175g of plain flour/ all-purpose flour, and mix together.
4. Add in 115g of cold butter to the mixing bowl and mix the ingredients together with your hands.
5. Add a generous even layer of crumble topping to the top of the raspberries.
6. Place the ovenproof dish in the oven and bake until the top of the crumble turns golden brown, for approximately 30 minutes.
7. Serve.

*Top Tip

Serve this raspberry crumble with some custard or vanilla ice cream.

Apple Flapjacks

Ingredients
- 2 Red Apples
- 425g Porridge Oats
- 250g Caster Sugar
- 180g Golden Syrup
- 250g Butter

Method

1. Preheat the oven to 180c/ gas mark 4 and line either a cake tin or an oven proof dish with baking paper.
2. Add 250g of butter to a large saucepan and place over a medium heat.
3. Add in 250g of caster sugar and 180g of golden syrup, stir until all of the sugar has dissolved.
4. Remove the saucepan from the heat and stir in 425g of porridge oats.
5. Peel and chop 2 red apples into small fine pieces, discard any pips, core, and skin.
6. Add the apple pieces into the saucepan and stir well.
7. Pour the ingredients out into the cake tin and smooth the top as you spread it out evenly.
8. Place the cake tin the oven and bake for 30 minutes.
9. Allow the flapjack to cool before cutting it into even bars.
10. Serve.

*Top Tip

If the flapjack becomes too moist, you can try grating the apple into the oats.

Banana Bread

Ingredients
- 2 Ripe Bananas
- 2 Eggs
- 140g Butter
- 140g Caster Sugar
- 140g Self Raising Flour
- 1 Teaspoon Baking Powder

Banana Icing
- 60g Butter
- 125g Mashed Banana
- ½ Teaspoon Lemon Juice
- ½ Teaspoon Vanilla Extract
- 400-500g Icing Sugar

Method

1. Preheat the oven to 180c/ gas mark 4.
2. Grease a loaf tin with a little bit of butter and then line with a sheet of greaseproof paper.
3. Place 140g of butter and 170g of sugar in a large mixing bowl and cream the ingredients together until they become light and fluffy.
4. Gradually add in 2 eggs with some of the self-raising flour.
5. Fold in the remaining flour and mix well.
6. Add in 1 teaspoon of baking powder.
7. Mash 2 ripe bananas in a separate bowl and then add them to the mixing bowl.
8. Stir the ingredients together.
9. Pour the mixture out into the loaf tin and place in the oven.

10. Bake for 30-40 minutes, or until a skewer comes out of the bread clean without any mixture stuck to it.
11. Leave the banana bread to cool for at least 10 minutes before transferring it to a wire rack.
12. Place 60g of butter and 125g of mashed banana in a bowl and cream together.
13. Add ½ teaspoon of lemon juice and ½ teaspoon of vanilla extract to the bowl and mix together.
14. Slowly beat in 400g-500g of icing sugar. Beat until the icing becomes nice and fluffy.
15. Cover the top of the banana loaf with a generous layer of banana icing.
16. Serve.

*Top Tip

If you prefer vanilla icing, you can add that to the top of the banana bread instead of the banana icing. Alternatively, you can serve the banana bread without any icing on top at all.

Apricot Squares

Ingredients
- 115g Plain Flour
- 115g Butter
- 55g Caster Sugar

Topping
- 140g Dried Apricots
- 170g Brown Sugar
- 55g Plain Flour
- 2 Eggs
- ½ Teaspoon of Vanilla Essence
- ¼ Teaspoon Salt
- 1 Tablespoon of Icing Sugar

Method

1. Preheat the oven to 180c/ gas mark 4.
2. Grease and line a shallow square baking tin.
3. Add 115g of butter and 55g of caster to a large mixing bowl and cream together until light and fluffy.
4. Gradually add in 115g of plain flour. Stir the ingredients together until a crumbly mixture is created.
5. Add the mixture to the baking tin and spread out evenly. Press and smooth the top with the back of a spoon.
6. Place the baking tin in the oven and bake for 25 minutes.
7. Place140g of dried apricots in a medium sized saucepan and cover with fresh cold water. Place the lid on top of the saucepan and cook over a medium heat for approximately 15 minutes.

8. Remove the saucepan from the heat and drain the apricots.
9. Chop the apricots up into small fine pieces.
10. Add 170g of brown sugar and 55g of plain flour to a mixing bowl.
11. Beat 2 eggs in a small bowl and then pour in over the brown sugar and plain flour.
12. Add the apricots to the mixing bowl along with ½ teaspoon of vanilla essence and ¼ teaspoon of salt and mix together.
13. Pour the topping mixture out directly on top of the biscuit base and evenly spread and smooth it out.
14. Place the baking tin back in the oven and bake for a further 25 minutes.
15. Leave to cool down in the tin for at least 10 minutes before cutting it up into apricot squares.
16. Sprinkle 1 tablespoon of icing sugar over the top.
17. Serve.

Pineapple, Carrot & Sultana Muffins

Ingredients
- 100g Plain Flour
- 100g Plain Wholemeal Flour
- 75g Caster Sugar
- 125g Carrot, Grated
- 225g Tinned Pineapple
- 100g Sultanas
- 4floz Rapeseed Oil
- 2 Eggs
- 1 Teaspoon Baking Powder
- ¾ Teaspoon Bicarbonate Soda
- 1 Teaspoon Ground Cinnamon
- 1 Teaspoon Ground Ginger
- 1 Tablespoon Rapeseed Oil
- ½ Teaspoon Salt

Method

1. Preheat the oven to 180c/ gas mark 4. Line a muffin tray with paper cases.
2. Sift 100g of plain flour and 100g of plain wholemeal flour in a medium sized mixing bowl.
3. Add 1 teaspoon of baking powder, ¾ teaspoon of bicarbonate soda, 1 teaspoon of ginger and 1 teaspoon of cinnamon to the flour and stir well.
4. Add ½ teaspoon of salt into the mixing bowl and stir.
5. Beat 2 eggs in a large mixing bowl.
6. Add 4floz of rapeseed oil to the eggs and 75g of caster sugar. Beat the ingredients together.
7. Add in 125g of grated carrot to the egg mixture, along with 225g of canned pineapple and 100g of Sultanas. Blend the ingredients together.

8. Gradually add in the flour mixture and stir well.
9. Evenly pour out the mixture into the muffin cases.
10. Place the muffin tray in the oven and bake for 25 minutes or until the muffins are golden brown.
11. Remove the muffins from the tray and leave to cool on a wire rack.
12. Serve.

*Top Tip

If you prefer to use fairy cake tins, reduce the cooking time by up to ten minutes to ensure that they do not burn.

Creamy Rice Pudding

Ingredients

- 120g Pudding Rice
- 800ml Milk
- 200ml of Water
- 4 Tablespoons of Maple Syrup
- 1 Vanilla Pod

Method

1. Place 120g of pudding rice in a large saucepan.
2. Cover the rice with 800ml of milk and 200ml of water.
3. Place the saucepan over a low heat.
4. Add 2 tablespoons of maple syrup to the saucepan and the vanilla. Stir well.
5. Cook the rice pudding until it becomes thick and creamy for approximately 40-45 minutes, making sure that you stir the ingredients regularly.
6. Remove from the heat and divide the rice pudding into individual bowls.
7. Drizzle the remaining maple syrup over the rice puddings.
8. Serve.

*Top Tip

You can substitute the maple syrup with honey if you prefer. You can also try adding various fruits to the rice pudding such as blueberries and raspberries. Alternatively, you can add a little cocoa powder to the ingredients to create a chocolate rice pudding.

Fruit Shortbread

Ingredients
- 750g Plain Flour
- 500g Margarine
- 250g Caster Sugar
- 110g Dried Cranberries
- 2 Orange Zests

Method

1. Preheat the oven to 140c/ gas mark 1 and line a baking tray with greaseproof paper.
2. Place 500g of margarine and 250g of caster sugar in a large mixing bowl and cream together until light and fluffy.
3. Sieve in 750g of plain flour and mix together.
4. Add in 100g of dried cranberries and 2 orange zests.
5. Mix the ingredients together to form a dough.
6. Pour the mixture out into the baking tray. Smooth and spread it out evenly.
7. Place the baking tray in the oven and bake for 35-40 minutes.
8. Allow the shortbread to cool down on the baking tray before cutting it up into squares.
9. Serve.

*Top Tip

You can substitute the dried cranberries for alternative fruits such as apricots, raisins, raspberries, sultanas, etc.

Bread & Butter Pudding

Ingredients
- 400ml Milk
- 100g Caster Sugar
- 100g Butter
- 5-10 Slices Bread
- 4 Eggs
- 1 Teaspoon Ground Cinnamon
- 1 Teaspoon Vanilla Essence

Method

1. Preheat the oven to 180c/gas mark 4.
2. Lightly grease a shallow ovenproof dish.
3. Spread the butter over both sides of the bread slices.
4. Add 100g of caster sugar to a mixing bowl along with 1 teaspoon of ground cinnamon. Mix the ingredients together.
5. Cut the slices of bread diagonally to create triangles and then layer the shallow ovenproof dish with the bread slices.
6. Pour 400ml of milk into a large mixing bowl and beat in 4 eggs. Add in 1 teaspoon of vanilla essence and stir in the sugar.
7. Pour the milk mixture over the bread triangles. Allow the bread slices to soak in the liquid for 20-30 minutes.
8. Place the ovenproof dish in the oven and bake for 25-30 minutes or until the pudding has set and browned.
9. Serve.

*Top Tip

You can add some sultanas to this recipe to make it a little fruitier.

Carrot Cake

Ingredients

- 225g Self-raising Flour
- 225g Carrots, Peeled and Grated
- 225g Fromage Frais
- 100g Soft Brown Sugar
- 90ml Sunflower Oil
- 50g Icing Sugar
- 4 Tablespoons Honey
- 2 Eggs
- 2 Tablespoon Lemon Juice
- 1 Teaspoon Ground Cinnamon

Method

1. Preheat the oven to 180c/gas mark 4.
2. Lightly grease a loaf tin with some butter and line with a sheet of greaseproof paper.
3. Sift 225g of self-raising flour into a large mixing bowl.
4. Add 1 teaspoon of ground cinnamon to the flour.
5. In another large mixing bowl crack and beat 2 eggs. Add in 4 tablespoons of honey, 90ml sunflower oil and 100g of soft brown sugar. Mix the ingredients together well before adding in 225g of peeled and grated carrots and 1 tablespoon of lemon juice.
6. Mix the carrot mixture into the flour until the ingredients are well combined.
7. Spoon the ingredients into the loaf tin and smooth the surface with the back of a spoon or with a clean knife.
8. Place the loaf tin in the oven and bake for 25-30 minutes, or until a skewer inserted into the center of the cake comes out clean.

9. Allow the carrot cake to cool down a little before removing it from the loaf tin and placing it on a wire rack.
10. In a medium sized mixing bowl add 225g of fromage frais, 50g of icing sugar and 1 tablespoon of lemon juice. Mix the ingredients together until they are well combined.
11. Ice the top of the carrot cake with the icing.
12. Serve.

Pineapple & Raisin Pudding

Ingredients
- 125g Self-Raising Flour
- 125g Margarine
- 100g Caster Sugar
- 3 Eggs
- 75g Crushed Pineapple Chunks, drained
- 75g Raisins
- 25g Cocoa Powder

Method

1. Preheat the oven to 180c/ gas mark 4. Grease a sandwich tin.
2. Add 125g of margarine and 100g of caster sugar to a large mixing bowl and cream together.
3. Beat in the eggs one at a time.
4. Add 25g of cocoa powder to the ingredients.
5. Gradually sieve 125g of self-raising flour into the mixing bowl and stir.
6. Fold in 75g of crushed pineapple chunks and 75g of raisins. Mix the ingredients together well.
7. Pour the mixture out into the sandwich tin and place in the center of the oven. Bake for 18-20 minutes, or until the center of the pudding becomes springy.
8. Allow the pudding to cool before transferring it to a wire rack or a plate.
9. Divide the pudding up into equal pieces.
10. Serve.

*Top Tip

You can serve this pudding with either vanilla custard or chocolate custard.

Fruit Scones

Ingredients

- 1kg Self-Raising Flour
- 250g Unsaturated Margarine
- 250g Sugar
- 200ml Milk
- 150g Sultanas
- 3 Eggs

Method

1. Preheat the oven to 180c/ gas mark 4.
2. Sieve 1kg of self-raising flour into a large mixing bowl and add in 250g of unsaturated margarine. Rub the ingredients together until it resembles small breadcrumbs.
3. Add 250g of sugar to the mixing bowl, followed by 200ml of milk and mix together.
4. Beat 3eggs in a small bowl and add them to the ingredients.
5. Add 150g of sultanas to the mixing bowl and stir together to form a dough.
6. Transfer the dough to a clean and lightly floured worktop surface, using a rolling pin roll the dough out.
7. Cut out the scones with a 2" cutter.
8. Brush the tops of the scones with a little bit of milk and place on a baking tray. Bake in the oven for 15-20 minutes.
9. Place the scones on a wire rack and leave to cool.
10. Serve.

*Top Tip

These fruity scones taste delicious with some butter and homemade fruity jam. You can substitute the sultanas for apricots.

Ginger Pudding

Ingredients
- 125g Margarine
- 125g Caster Sugar
- 125g Ground Rice
- 100g Preserved Ginger
- 15ml Milk
- 2 Eggs

Method

1. Preheat the oven to 120c/ gas mark 2. Lightly oil a loaf tin and line with some baking paper.
2. Place 125g of margarine and 125g of caster sugar in a large mixing bowl and cream together.
3. Add in 125g of ground rice, 100g of preserved ginger (finely chopped) and 15ml of milk to the ingredients.
4. Beat the eggs into the mixture one at a time. Mix the ingredients together well.
5. Pour the pudding mixture into the loaf tin and place in the oven. Bake for 1½-2 hours, or until the center of the pudding is firm to the touch.
6. Allow the pudding to stand for at least 10-15 minutes before transferring it to a wire rack.
7. Serve.

*Top Tip

This ginger pudding tastes delicious with some vanilla custard.

Oat & Raisin Cookies

Ingredients
- 175g Plain Flour
- 125g Raisins
- 100g Margarine
- 75g Caster Sugar
- 75g Brown Sugar
- 75g Oats, Pre-toasted
- 1 Egg
- 1 Teaspoon of Vanilla Essence

Method

1. Preheat the oven to 180c/ gas mark 4. Grease 3 baking trays and line with baking paper.
2. Add 100g of margarine to a large mixing bowl and add in 75g of caster sugar and 75g of brown sugar. Cream the ingredients together.
3. Beat in the egg.
4. Gradually sieve in 175g of plain flour and fold into the creamed ingredients.
5. Add 75g of pre-toasted oats and 1 teaspoon of vanilla essence to the mixing bowl and mix well.
6. Using a spoon, heap the mixture into approximately 5cm individual cookies and spread apart on the baking trays.
7. Place the baking trays in the oven and bake for 12-15 minutes or until the cookies are lightly browned.
8. Remove the cookies from the baking trays and allow the cookies to cool down on a wire rack.
9. Serve.

*Top Tip

You can substitute the raisins with other dried fruit such as sultanas, cranberries, and apricots.

Custard

Ingredients

- 700ml Whole Milk
- 200ml Double Cream
- 200g Caster Sugar
- 4 Egg Yolks
- 3 Tablespoons Cornflour
- 1-2 Teaspoons Vanilla Extract.

Method

1. Pour 700ml of whole milk into a large saucepan and place over a low/medium heat.
2. Add 200ml of double cream to the milk and gently bring to just below boiling point.
3. Beat 4 egg yolks in a mixing bowl and add in 3 tablespoons of corn flour, 200g of caster sugar and 1-2 teaspoons of vanilla extract. Mix well.
4. Gradually pour the hot milk mixture into the mixing bowl, ensuring that you are constantly whisking the ingredients together.
5. Pour all of the ingredients into a large saucepan and place over a low heat.
6. Stir the custard with a wooden spoon until it has thickened.
7. Serve hot or cold.

*Top Tip

You can add a little bit of cocoa powder to the mixture to create a chocolate custard.

Snacks & Sides

Apple & Cinnamon Chips

Ingredients

- 3 Large Apples
- 2 Teaspoons of Cinnamon
- 1 Teaspoon of Fresh Cold Water
- 15g of Butter

Method

1. Preheat the oven to 180c/ gas mark 5.
2. Peel 3 large apples with a peeler or a knife and disregard the skin. Chop the apples up into long chunky individual pieces. Place the apples in a large mixing bowl.
3. Add 15g of butter in with the apple chunks, 2 teaspoons of cinnamon and 1 teaspoon of fresh cold water. Mix the ingredients together, blending well so that all of the apple chunks are coated.
4. Cover a large baking tray with a layer of greaseproof paper.
5. Place the apple chunks on top of the baking tray, spread them out and do not place the apples on top of each other.
6. Place the baking tray inside of the oven and bake for 15-20 minutes each side.
7. Leave to cool and serve warm.

*Top Tip

Serve the cinnamon apple fries in a glass, cone or on a plate.

Chocolate Strawberries

Ingredients
- 500g Strawberries
- 500g Milk Chocolate
- 2 Tablespoons of Butter

Method

1. Insert skewers into the tops of all of the strawberries.
2. Break up 500g of milk chocolate and place it inside a glass heatproof bowl. Add the glass bowl to a saucepan full of cold water and place over a low/medium heat.
3. Add 2 tablespoons of butter to the chocolate and stir until all of the chocolate and butter has melted and become smooth.
4. Dip the strawberries into the melted chocolate mixture by holding the skewers.
5. Turn the strawberries upside down and insert the skewers into a Styrofoam, or a potato. Allow the chocolate to cool and set for approximately 45-60 minutes.
6. Serve.

*Top Tip

You can add a layer of sprinkles after you have dipped the strawberries in melted chocolate.

Fruit Granola Bars

Ingredients
- 200g Oats
- 100g Butter
- 100g Brown Sugar
- 100g Dried Cranberries, Blueberries & Cherries
- 80g Sunflower Seeds
- 60g Sesame Seeds
- 40g Walnuts, Chopped
- 1 Tablespoons of Cinnamon
- 3 Tablespoons of Honey

Method

1. Preheat the oven to 160c/ gas mark 3 and line a baking tin approximately 18cm x 25cm with greaseproof paper.
2. Place 200g of oats in the baking tin along with 80g sunflower seeds, 60g sesame seeds and 40g of chopped walnuts and mix together.
3. Place the baking tin in the oven for 8-10 minutes until toasted.
4. Add 100g of butter to a saucepan and place over a medium/high heat until the butter has melted.
5. Add 3 tablespoons of honey and 100g of brown sugar to the saucepan and stir together.
6. Remove the oats from the oven.
7. Stir the toasted oat mix into the saucepan.
8. Add 1 tablespoon of cinnamon and 100g of dried fruit to the saucepan and stir until all of the oats are coated.

9. Empty the ingredients out into the baking tin and smooth out the top. Place the tin in the oven and cook for 25-30 minutes.
10. Allow to cool in the tin before cutting it up into 12 even bars.

*Top Tip

You can experiment with your fruit granola bars by adding different blends of fruit to the oat mixture such as raspberries, apricots, strawberries, and sultanas, etc.

Grilled Cheese & Spinach, Pepper Sandwich

Ingredients
- 2 Slices of Bread
- 60g of Cheddar Cheese
- 60g Havarti Cheese
- ½ Roasted Red Pepper
- A Handful of Fresh Spinach Leafs

Method

1. Layer one-half of the cheddar and Havarti cheese on a slice of bread.
2. Chop ½ roasted red pepper up into small pieces.
3. Add one layer of roasted red pepper to the top of the cheese.
4. Add 1 handful of fresh spinach leafs to the top of the red pepper.
5. Add the remaining pieces of cheese to the top of the spinach leafs and then cover with the last slice of bread.
6. Place the sandwich on a grill and cook until the bread goes golden brown, for approximately 4-5 minutes. Flip the sandwich over and cook for a further 4-5 minutes until the cheese in the middle has melted.
7. Serve hot.

*Top Tip

If you prefer to grill your sandwich on a griddle or in a heated skillet, lightly spread some butter on the outside of the sandwich before placing it on the heat.

Homemade Peanut Butter

Ingredients
- 600g of Dry Roasted Peanuts
- 2 Tablespoons of Honey

Method

1. Add 600g of dry roasted peanuts to a blender or a food processor. Blend the peanuts for 4-5 minutes, until they turn creamy.
2. Add 2 Tablespoons of honey to the blender and blend for a further 1 minute.
3. Scoop the peanut butter out into a clean empty jar and store at room temperature or in a refrigerator.

*Top Tip

The peanut butter can be kept in the refrigerator for several weeks. However, if you think that you will go through it faster, then you can store it at room temperature.

Lactation Cookies

Ingredients
- 255g of Oats
- 128g of Caster Sugar
- 227g of Butter
- 128g Brown Sugar
- 125g Milk Chocolate chips
- 4 Tablespoons of Water
- 2 Tablespoons of Flaxseed
- 1 Tablespoon of Vanilla Essence
- 2 Eggs
- 2 Tablespoons of Brewer's Yeast
- 1 Teaspoon of Baking Soda
- 1 Teaspoon of Salt

Method

1. Preheat the oven to 170c/ gas mark 3 and line a baking tray with greaseproof paper.
2. Add 2 tablespoons of flaxseed and 4 tablespoons of water to a small bowl, set aside for 4-5 minutes.
3. Add 227g of butter, 128g of caster sugar and 125g of brown sugar to a large mixing bowl and cream the ingredients together.
4. Crack 2 eggs into the mixing bowl and stir well.
5. Stir the flaxseed mixture into the mixing bowl.
6. Add 1 tablespoon of vanilla essence to the ingredients and stir well for 1-2 minutes.
7. Add 2 tablespoons of brewer's yeast, 1 teaspoon of baking soda and 1 teaspoon of salt to the mixing bowl.
8. Stir in 255g of oats and 125g of milk chocolate chips. Blend all of the ingredients together.

9. Equally, divide the cookie dough up into small round balls and place them onto a baking tray. Spread the cookies out and press them flat with a fork.
10. Place the baking tray in the oven and bake for 10-12 minutes.

*Top Tip

Instead of baking all of the cookies at once you can set aside half of the cookie dough and freeze it in the freezer and bake at a later date.

Pineapple Cinnamon Strips

Ingredients

- 1 Pineapple
- 2 Tablespoons of Cinnamon
- 60g of Honey

Method

1. Cut 1 pineapple up into long chunky strips.
2. Grill the pineapple strips for 5 minutes on a medium heat.
3. Place 60g of honey and 2 tablespoons of cinnamon in a small bowl and mix together.
4. Drizzle the grilled pineapple with the honey mixture and place back on the grill for a further 5-8 minutes.
5. Serve.

*Top Tip

If you prefer not to use honey, you could swap this ingredient with 25g of butter to mix with the cinnamon.

Stuffed Peppers

Ingredients
- 2 Large Red Peppers
- 85g Couscous
- 30g Pine Nuts
- 50g Feta Cheese
- 50g Cherry Tomatoes
- 125g Boiling Water
- A Small Handful of Black Olives, Pitted
- 2 Tablespoons of Shredded Fresh Basil

Method

1. Preheat the oven to 200c/ gas mark 6.
2. Slice 2 red peppers in half and deseed them. Place the red peppers onto a plate and microwave on a medium heat for 4-5 minutes, until they soften.
3. Place the red peppers onto a baking tray.
4. Add 85g of couscous to a medium sized bowl and pour in 125g of boiling water. Stir the ingredients together, cover the bowl and leave to stand for 10 whole minutes.
5. Chop 50g of cherry tomatoes up into small pieces.
6. Stir the couscous to break it up and then mix in 30g of pine nuts, a small handful of pitted black olives, 50g of feta cheese broken up, tomatoes and 2 tablespoons of shredded fresh basil. Stir the ingredients together and then spoon the couscous mixture into the peppers halves.
7. Place the baking tray in the oven and bake for 10-12 minutes.

*Top Tip

You can add a few chilies into the couscous mixture.

Spicy Sweet Potato Chips

Ingredients

- 2 Large Sweet Potatoes
- 3 Tablespoons of Rapeseed Oil
- 1 Teaspoon of Paprika
- 1 Teaspoon of Hot Curry Powder

Method

1. Preheat the oven to 190c /gas mark 5.
2. Peel 2 large sweet potatoes and discard the skin. Cut the sweet potato up into wedges and place in a large mixing bowl.
3. Add 3 Tablespoons of rapeseed oil to the sweet potatoes, 1 teaspoon of paprika and 1 teaspoon of hot curry powder. Stir the ingredients together.
4. Cover a baking tray with a sheet of greaseproof paper.
5. Place the sweet potato chips onto the baking tray and cook until crisp, for approximately 25-30 minutes depending on how thick your wedges have been cut. Turn the sweet potatoes over once half way through.

*Top Tip

Don't layer the sweet potatoes on top of each other when putting them in the oven.

Seasoned Yorkshire Puddings

Ingredients

- 250g Plain Flour
- 300ml Whole Milk
- 4 Eggs
- 6 Tablespoons of Rapeseed Oil
- 1 Teaspoon of Thyme
- 2 Teaspoons of Sage
- A Pinch of Salt

Method

1. Preheat the oven to 200c/ gas mark 6.
2. Sieve 250g of plain flour into a large mixing bowl.
3. Add 1 teaspoon of thyme, 2 teaspoons of sage and a pinch of salt to the flour and stir the ingredients together.
4. Make a well in the middle of the mixing bowl and gradually whisk in 300ml of whole milk and 4 eggs.
5. Whisk the ingredients for 6-8 minutes until a smooth batter is formed.
6. Pour 6 tablespoons of rapeseed oil into a roasting tin or equally into a 12 hole Yorkshire pudding tray.
7. Place the roasting tin in the oven and leave the oil to heat for 15-20 minutes.
8. Once the oil is boiling, pour the batter into the roasting tin, or into the 12 Yorkshire pudding holes so that they are half way full.
9. Place the roasting tin back inside of the oven and cook for 15-20 minutes, or until the Yorkshire puddings have risen and turned golden brown.
10. Serve.

*Top Tip

You can add more or less seasoning to match your personal tastes. You can also experiment with different seasonings by adding different flavours such as pepper, chives, onion, etc.

Seasoned Vegetables

Ingredients

- ½ Butternut Squash
- 1 Sweet Potato
- 3 Carrots
- 150g Brussel Sprouts
- 2 Parsnips
- 3 Tablespoons of Rapeseed Oil
- ¾ Teaspoon of Kosher Salt
- ¾ Teaspoon of Ground Black Pepper
- 4 Garlic Cloves
- 1 Teaspoon of Rosemary

Method

1. Preheat the oven to 190c/ gas mark 5.
2. Peel and chop ½ butternut squash, 1 sweet potato, 3 carrots and 2 parsnips into small chunky pieces and place in an ovenproof dish or a roasting tray.
3. Add 150g of Brussel sprouts to the vegetables.
4. In a small bowl add 3 tablespoons of rapeseed oil, ¾ teaspoon of kosher salt, ¾ teaspoon of ground black pepper, 4 chopped cloves of garlic and 1 teaspoon of rosemary and mix together.
5. Drizzle the oil mixture over the vegetables and toss the oven proof dish, ensuring all of the vegetables are coated.
6. Place the ovenproof dish in the oven and cook for approximately 40-45 minutes, stirring the vegetables halfway through.

*Top Tip

You can try adding a wide variety of vegetables to this dish including cauliflower florets, broccoli, mushrooms, onions, etc. to suit your personal taste.

Mediterranean Vegetables

Ingredients

- 350g Potatoes
- 250g Cherry Tomatoes
- 1 Eggplant
- 1 Red Pepper
- 1 Green Pepper
- 1 Red Onion
- 1 Courgette
- 3 Tablespoons of Rapeseed Oil
- 1 Teaspoon of Basil
- 1 Teaspoon of Oregano
- 1 Teaspoon of Chives
- 5 Garlic Cloves
- ¼ Teaspoon of Kosher Salt
- ¼ Teaspoon of Ground Black Pepper

Method

1. Preheat the oven to 190c/ gas mark 5.
2. Peel 350g of potatoes and chop them into halves and then into quarters. Place the potatoes in a large ovenproof dish or in a roasting tray.
3. Chop 1 eggplant and 1 courgette up into small chunky pieces and add to the potatoes.
4. Chop and deseed 1 red pepper and 1 green pepper and add to the ovenproof dish.
5. Peel 1 red onion and chop it into small pieces. Add the onion to the potatoes.
6. Add 250g of cherry tomatoes to the ovenproof dish and stir the ingredients.
7. Add 3 tablespoons of rapeseed oil to a small bowl, followed by 1 teaspoon of basil, 1 teaspoon of

oregano, 1 teaspoon of chives, ¼ teaspoon of kosher salt, ¼ teaspoon of ground black pepper and 5 cloves of chopped garlic. Whisk the ingredients together until they are well blended.

8. Drizzle the oil mixture over the vegetables and toss the oven proof dish, ensuring all of the vegetables are coated.

9. Place the ovenproof dish in the oven and cook for approximately 45 minutes, stirring the vegetables halfway through.

*Top Tip

This recipe is a perfect side dish for chicken, steak or fish meals.

Parmesan Straws

Ingredients

- 125g Butter
- 125g Plain Flour
- 85g Parmesan Cheese
- ¼ Teaspoon Salt
- ¼ Teaspoon Ground Black Pepper
- 4 Tablespoons of Milk

Method

1. Preheat the oven to 180c/ gas mark 4.
2. Add 125g of Butter to a large mixing bowl.
3. Add 85g of parmesan cheese to the butter and beat together until they are well blended.
4. Sieve 125g of plain flour into the mixing bowl.
5. Add ¼ teaspoon of salt, and ¼ teaspoon of ground black pepper to the ingredients and stir together until a dough has formed.
6. Divide the dough into half and place it on a clean, lightly floured surface.
7. Using a rolling pin, roll out each of the portions into approximately 45x7cm rectangles and then cut into 7x1cm strips.
8. Cover a baking tray with greaseproof paper and then place the individual strips 2cm apart on the baking tray.
9. Brush the straw strips with 4 tablespoons of milk.
10. Place the baking tray in the oven and bake for 8-10 minutes, or until the straws are lightly browned.
11. Leave to cool and then serve.

Cheesy Chili Relleno Squares

Ingredients
- 200g Cheddar Cheese
- 200g Red Leicester Cheese
- 3 Green Chili Peppers
- 2 Eggs
- 2 Tablespoons of Milk
- 1 Tablespoon of All Purpose Flour

Method

1. Preheat the oven to 190c /gas mark 5.
2. Cut 3 green chili peppers open lengthways and remove the seeds. Rinse with fresh cold water.
3. Place 200g of Cheddar Cheese in a large mixing bowl and add in 200g of red Leicester cheese. Mix the two kinds of cheese together.
4. Crack 2 eggs into the mixing bowl and mix with the cheese.
5. Add 1 tablespoon of milk and 1 tablespoon of all-purpose flour to the mixing bowl and stir the ingredients together until smooth.
6. Grease an oven proof dish or layer it with greaseproof paper.
7. Chop the green chili peppers up into small pieces and add to the mixing bowl. Stir well.
8. Pour the cheesy mixture out into the greased ovenproof dish, making sure it is evenly spread out.
9. Place the ovenproof dish in the oven and back uncovered for 50 minutes, or until golden.
10. Serve hot or cold.

Rosemary Roast Potatoes

Ingredients
- 600g of White Potato
- 18g Rapeseed Oil
- 1 Teaspoon of Ground Black Pepper
- ¾ Teaspoon of Kosher Salt
- 5 Cloves of Garlic
- 3 Tablespoons of Finely Chopped Fresh Rosemary Leaves
- 1 Onion.

Method

1. Preheat the oven to 190c/ gas mark 5.
2. Peel 600g of white potatoes, chop them in halves and then into quarters.
3. Place the potatoes in either a large oven proof dish or in a roasting tray.
4. Drip 18g of rapeseed oil over the potatoes.
5. Sprinkle 1 teaspoon of ground black pepper, ¾ teaspoon of kosher salt and 3 tablespoons of finely chopped fresh rosemary leaves on top of the potatoes.
6. Add five cloves of garlic to the ovenproof dish, making sure that they are spread apart.
7. Peel 1 onion and chop into small wedges. Add the onion to the oven proof dish in between the potatoes.
8. Toss the oven proof dish until the potatoes are well coated with the ingredients.
9. Place the ovenproof dish in the oven and cook for at least one hour, making sure that you turn the potatoes halfway through. Cook until the potatoes have browned and turned crisp.
10. Serve.

*Top Tip

You can add more seasoning to this recipe to suit your individual taste.

Bread

Cloud Bread

Ingredients

- 200g Cheddar Cheese
- 3Eggs, Separated
- 55g Soft Cream Cheese
- ¼ Teaspoon Cream of Tartar
- 1 Tablespoon Sugar

Method

1. Preheat the oven to 180c/ Gas Mark 4. Line a baking tray with a sheet of baking paper.
2. Add ¼ teaspoon of cream of tartar to the egg whites and beat together in a small bowl until stiff peaks start to form.
3. In a separate bowl, add the egg yolks, 55g of soft cream cheese and 1 tablespoon of sugar. Mix the ingredients together until the mixture becomes smooth and the cream cheese is no longer visible.
4. Gently fold in the egg white mixture into the egg yolks. Take your time and be careful not to deflate the egg whites.
5. Using your hands, carefully form 6 equal bun shapes. Place each of the buns on the baking tray making sure you space them out.
6. Place the baking tray in the oven and cook for 25-30 minutes, or until the cloud bread has lightly browned.

Soda Bread

Ingredients
- 170g Self-Raising Wholemeal Flour
- 170g Plain Flour
- 290ml Buttermilk
- ½ Teaspoon Salt
- ½ Teaspoon Bicarbonate of Soda

Method

1. Preheat the oven to 200c/gas mark 6. Line a baking tray with a sheet of baking paper.
2. Pour 170g of self-raising wholemeal flour into a large mixing bowl along with 170g of plain flour, ½ teaspoon of salt and ½ teaspoon of bicarbonate of soda and stir the ingredients together.
3. Make a well in the center of the flour and pour in 290ml of buttermilk. Swiftly mix the ingredients together with a large wooden spoon to form a soft dough.
4. Lightly flour a clean worktop surface and place the dough on top. Knead the dough for 3-4 minutes.
5. Form the dough into a round dome and lightly flatten with the palm of your hand.
6. Lightly flour the sheet of baking paper and place the dough on top.
7. Cut a cross on top of the dough with a knife.
8. Place the baking tray in the oven and bake for 30 minutes, or until the loaf sounds hollow when tapped.
9. Cool the sofa bread on a wire rack.
10. Slice and serve.

Garlic Bread

Ingredients

- 4 Cloves of Garlic
- 110g of Butter
- 2 Tablespoons of Extra Rapeseed Oil
- 1 Loaf of Italian Bread/Baguette
- 30g Grated Parmigiano/ Mozzarella
- ½ Teaspoon Fresh Parsley, Chopped

Method

1. Preheat the oven to 180c/ gas mark 4. Line a baking tray with a sheet of baking paper.
2. Add 2 tablespoons of butter to a medium sized saucepan and place over a medium heat.
3. Chop or mince 4 cloves of garlic into small pieces.
4. Once the butter has melted, add the garlic to the saucepan and ½ teaspoon of chopped fresh parsley.
5. Cut the Italian bread or baguette up into ½ inch slices. Place the Italian bread on the baking paper.
6. Use a basting brush to brush the slices of bread with the butter mixture generously.
7. Place the baking tray in the oven and cook for 8-10 minutes, or until the bread is slightly toasted.
8. Remove the baking tray from the oven and sprinkle the slices of bread with the grated Parmigiano/mozzarella cheese and any remaining butter mixture.
9. Return the baking tray back in the oven and cook for a further 5-6 minutes, or until the cheese has melted and the bread has slightly browned.
10. Serve.

*Top Tip

This garlic bread tastes delicious with pasta dishes.

Sesame Seed Bread Rolls

Ingredients

- 500g Strong Plain White Flour
- 30g of Butter
- 75ml of Warmed Whole Milk
- 225ml Lukewarm Water
- 1 Teaspoon of Sugar
- 1 Teaspoon of Salt
- 2 Teaspoons of Dried Yeast
- 3 Tablespoons of Sesame Seeds
- 1 Tablespoon of Whole Milk

Method

1. Sieve 500g of strong plain white flour into a large mixing bowl.
2. Add in 1 teaspoon of salt, and 2 teaspoons of dried yeast and stir together.
3. Rub 30g of butter into the flour mixture using your fingertips until it turns into breadcrumbs.
4. Pour 75ml of warmed whole milk into a jug and add in 225ml of lukewarm water. Pour the liquid into the flour mixture, mixing well with a large spoon until a soft dough is created.
5. Lightly flour a clean work surface and empty the dough onto it. Knead the dough for a good 15-20 minutes until it becomes stretchy and elastic.
6. Place the dough back inside of the large mixing bowl and cover it up with a damp tea towel. Leave the bowl in a warm, dry place for at least 1 hour so that it can rise.
7. Once the dough has doubled in size, remove the dough from the mixing bowl and knead for a couple

more minutes. Divide the dough up into 6 even portions and shape them into bread rolls.

8.   Place the bread rolls onto a slightly oiled baking tray, spacing them out. Cover the baking tray with some clingfilm and leave to prove in a warm, dry place for a further 1 hour, until the dough has doubled in size once again.

9.   Preheat the oven to 220c/ gas mark 7.

10.   Once the dough has doubled in size remove the clingfilm from the baking tray. With a knife, make a few incisions on the tops of the bread rolls.

11.   Place the baking tray in the oven and bake for 10-12 minutes until the bread rolls have turned golden and have risen.

12.   Place 1 tablespoon of milk and 1 teaspoon of sugar in a small bowl and mix together until the sugar has fully dissolved.

13.   Remove the bread rolls from the oven and brush the tops of them with the milk glaze.

14.   Equally, scatter the sesame seeds on top of the bread rolls so that they stick to the tops of the bread.

15.   Transfer the bread rolls onto a wire rack and leave to cool before serving.

Cheesy Garlic Bread

Ingredients
- 500g Strong White Bread Flour
- 300ml Hand-hot Water
- 100g Mature Cheddar Cheese, Grated
- 25g Soft Butter
- 7g Sachet/ 1½ Teaspoon Fast-action Yeast
- 4 Cloves of Garlic
- 2 Tablespoons of Rapeseed Oil
- 1 Teaspoon Salt
- 1 Tablespoon Clear Honey
- Handful of fresh Thyme Leaves

Method

1. Place 500g of strong white bread flour, 1½ teaspoons of fast-action yeast and 1 teaspoon of salt in a large mixing bowl.
2. Pour 300ml of hand hot water into a jug and add 1 tablespoon of clear honey and 2 tablespoons of rapeseed oil and stir together. Pour the liquid into the mixing bowl, constantly stirring to make a soft dough.
3. Lightly flour a clean worktop surface and place the dough on top. Knead the dough for 4-5 minutes until the dough no longer feels sticky. You can sprinkle a little more flour on top if you need it.
4. Stretch the dough out to fit a Swiss roll tin.
5. In a small bowl add 25g of soft butter and 4 crushed or chopped garlic cloves. Mix the ingredients together and then brush over the dough.
6. Sprinkle the dough with 100g of grated mature cheddar cheese.
7. Top the cheese with a handful of fresh thyme leaves.

8. Lightly oil a sheet of cling film and use this to cover up the bread. Leave to rise in a warm place for 40-50 minutes.
9. Heat the oven to 190c/ gas mark 5.
10. Remove the cling film from the dough and place the Swiss roll tin in the oven and bake for 30 minutes, or until the bread has risen and turned golden.
11. Leave to cool for 10-15 minutes.
12. Cut the bread up into 12 slices and serve.

*Top Tip

This garlic bread tastes delicious with pasta and salad dishes.

Focaccia with Pesto & Mozzarella

Ingredients
- 500g Strong White Bread Flour
- 325ml Tepid Water
- 125g Ball Mozzarella, Drained
- 7g Sachet/ 1½ Teaspoon Fast-action Yeast
- 5 Tablespoons Pesto
- 2 Tablespoons of Rapeseed Oil
- 1½ Teaspoon Salt
- Sea Salt (Optional)

Method

1. Place 500g of strong white bread flour in a large mixing bowl and mix in 1½ teaspoons of salt.
2. In a jug, mix 325ml of tepid water with 1½ teaspoons of fast-action yeast.
3. Add 2 tablespoons of rapeseed oil to the flour and pour in the water mixture. Mix the ingredients together with a large wooden spoon or with your hands. Use your hands to create one big ball of dough.
4. Lightly flour a clean worktop surface and place the dough on top. Knead the dough for 10-15 minutes, making sure you pull and stretch the dough out so that as much air can get to it as possible.
5. Oil a mixing bowl and a sheet of cling film. Place the ball of dough into the well-oiled mixing bowl and cover with the oiled sheet of cling film. Leave the dough to rise in a warm place for 50-60 minutes, until the dough has doubled in size.
6. Cover a baking tray with a sheet of baking paper.
7. Stretch the dough out onto the baking paper until it is about 20x30cm long.

8. Loosely cover the dough with a clean tea towel. Leave the dough to rise for a further 30-40 minutes in a warm place, until it rises to about half as high again.
9. Heat the oven to 180/ gas mark 4.
10. Once the dough has risen, press your fingers into it and gently make some holes.
11. Place the baking tray in the oven and bake for about 15 minutes before removing from the oven.
12. Cover the bread with 125g of mozzarella cheese and then place the baking tray back in the oven and bake for a further 5-10 minutes, or until the bread is golden and cooked through.
13. Remove the bread from the oven and drizzle with pesto and sea salt.
14. Slice and serve.

Sundried Tomato & Olive Bread

Ingredients

- 500g Strong White Flour
- 275ml Tepid Water
- 170g Black Olives, Pitted
- 55g Sun Dried Tomatoes
- 55ml Olive Oil
- 20g Fresh Yeast
- 15g Salt

Method

1. Place 500g of strong white flour in a large mixing bowl along with 15g of salt.
2. Add 275ml of tepid water to the flour, 55ml of olive oil and 20g of fresh yeast. Mix the ingredients together.
3. Knead well with your hands and knuckles until an elastic, smooth and shiny dough is formed.
4. Oil a sheet of cling film and cover the mixing bowl with it. Leave the dough in a warm place to rise for 50-60 minutes.
5. Divide the dough into two pieces.
6. Add half of the black olives and sun-dried tomatoes into each of the dough pieces.
7. Mold both of the doughs into round shapes and press down firmly using the palm of your hand.
8. Mark the tops of the dough with a cross and lightly sprinkle each one with some flour.
9. Line a baking tray with a sheet of baking paper and place the dough on top, making sure that they are spread apart. Prove for a further 50-60 minutes in a warm place.

10. Heat the oven to 220c/ gas mark 7.
11. Place the baking tray in the oven and bake for 25-30 minutes, or until the bread has turned golden-brown and cooked through.
12. Remove the bread from the oven and transfer to a wire rack. Leave to cool.
13. Slice and serve.

Rustic Rolls

Ingredients

- 500g Wholemeal Bread Flour
- 300ml Warm Water
- 7g Sachet/ 1½ Teaspoon Fast-action Yeast
- 2 Teaspoons of Salt
- 1½ Teaspoons of Sugar
- 1 Tablespoon of Butter
- 4 Tablespoons of Olive Oil

Method

1. Place 500g of wholemeal bread flour in a large mixing bowl along with 2 teaspoons of salt, 1½ teaspoons of sugar and 1½ teaspoons of fast-action yeast. Mix the ingredients together.
2. Make a well in the center of the flour.
3. In a jug add 300ml of warm water and 3 tablespoons of olive oil, mix the ingredients together.
4. Pour the water into the well and gradually mix together with the flour until a dough forms.
5. Lightly flour a clean worktop surface and place the dough on top. Knead the dough for 10-15 minutes, until the dough becomes smooth and elastic.
6. Oil a mixing bowl and a sheet of cling film.
7. Place the dough in the oiled mixing bowl and cover it up with the oiled sheet of cling film. Leave to prove in a warm place for 50-60 minutes.
8. Once the dough has risen knead for another 8-10 minutes, before rolling it out into a long sausage shape and dividing it up into 8 equal sections.
9. Form each of the sections into small rounded rolls and gently flatten with your palm.

10. Line a baking tray with a sheet of baking paper and place the bread rolls on top.
11. Cover the dough with a clean tea towel and leave to prove for another 60 minutes.
12. Heat the oven to 220c/ gas mark 7.
13. Remove the tea towel from the dough and place the baking tray in the oven. Bake for 12-15 minutes or until the bread has turned golden brown, cooked through and sounds hollow.
14. Remove the bread from the oven and transfer to a wire rack, leave to cool.
15. Lightly dust with some flour. Place a clean tea towel over the bread rolls while cooling to absorb the moisture.
16. Serve.

*Top Tip

These rustic bread rolls taste beautiful with some homemade soup.

Jams

Strawberry Jam

Ingredients
- 900g Strawberries
- 900g Golden Granulated Sugar
- 3 Tablespoons Lemon Juice
- Knob of Butter

Method

1. Wipe 900g of fresh raspberries with some clean damp kitchen paper.
2. Hull the fruit with a knife by cutting the strawberries into a cone shape and removing the stems. Cut any large strawberries in half.
3. Place the strawberries in a large saucepan and add in 900g of golden granulated sugar. Toss the ingredients together and leave uncovered at room temperature for several hours, or overnight.
4. Add 3 tablespoon of lemon juice to the strawberries and place the saucepan over a low/medium heat. Gently cook for 4-5 minutes until the fruit softens and the juice runs.
5. Once all of the sugar granules have dissolved increase the heat.
6. Bring to the boil and boil for a further 20-25 minutes. Don't stir the strawberries until the setting point is reached of 105c.
7. Remove the saucepan from the heat.
8. Spoon a little of the hot jam onto a chilled saucer or a small plate. Leave for a couple of minutes and then push your finger into the jam. If the jam wrinkles then it is ready, if the jam remains runny then return the

saucepan back to the heat and boil for a few more minutes before testing again.

9. Remove any scrum from the surface with a spoon.
10. Stir in a knob of butter across the jam surface, this will help to dissolve any remaining scum.
11. Leave to settle for about 10-15 minutes
12. Pour the hot jam into warm sterilised jars, seal and label.

Raspberry Jam

Ingredients
- 900g Fresh Raspberries
- 900g Preserving Sugar
- 1 Tablespoon Lemon Juice
- Knob of Butter

Method

1. Rinse 900g of fresh raspberries in cold water and then place them in a large saucepan.
2. Add 1 tablespoon of lemon juice to the raspberries and place the saucepan over a low/medium heat. Gently cook for 4-5 minutes until the fruit softens and the juice runs.
3. Add in 900g of preserving sugar to the fruit and stir together. Keep the saucepan over a low/medium heat until all of the sugar has dissolved.
4. Bring to the boil and boil for a further 10 minutes.
5. Remove the saucepan from the heat.
6. Spoon a little of the hot jam onto a chilled saucer or a small plate. Leave for a couple of minutes and then push your finger into the jam. If the jam wrinkles then it is ready, if the jam remains runny then return the saucepan back to the heat and boil for a few more minutes before testing again.
7. Remove any scrum from the surface with a spoon.
8. Stir in a knob of butter across the jam surface, this will help to dissolve any remaining scum.
9. Leave to settle for about 10-15 minutes
10. Pour the hot jam into warm sterilised jars, seal and label.

Blackberry Jam

Ingredients

- 900g Blackberries
- 900g Golden Granulated Sugar
- 50ml Water
- 1 ½ tablespoons of Lemon Juice
- Knob of Butter

Method

1. Rinse 900g of fresh blackberries in cold water and then place them in a large saucepan.
2. Pour 50ml of water into the saucepan and add in 1½ tablespoons of lemon juice.
3. Place the saucepan over a low/medium heat. Simmer the fruit for 15 minutes until the fruit softens, and the juice runs.
4. Add 900g of golden granulated sugar to the fruit and simmer on a low heat until all of the sugar has completely dissolved.
5. Increase the heat and bring to the boil. Boil, for a further 10-15 minutes.
6. Spoon a little of the hot jam onto a chilled saucer or a small plate. Leave for a couple of minutes and then push your finger into the jam. If the jam wrinkles then it is ready, if the jam remains runny then return the saucepan back to the heat and boil for a few more minutes before testing again.
7. Remove any scrum from the surface with a spoon.
8. Stir in a knob of butter across the jam surface; this will help to dissolve any remaining scum.
9. Leave the jam to settle for 10-15 minutes

10. Pour the hot jam into warm sterilised jars, seal and label.

Plum Jam

Ingredients
- 900g of Plums
- 900g Golden Granulated Sugar
- 150ml Water
- Knob of Butter

Method

1. Rinse 900g of fresh halved and stoned plums in cold water, and then place them in a large saucepan.
2. Pour 150ml of water into the saucepan and add in 1½ tablespoons of lemon juice.
3. Place the saucepan over a low/medium heat. Simmer the fruit for 30-40 minutes until the fruit softens and the juice runs.
4. Add in 900g of golden granulated sugar to the fruit and simmer on a low heat until all of the sugar has completely dissolved.
5. Increase the heat and bring to the boil. Boil for a further 10 minutes.
6. Spoon a little of the hot jam onto a chilled saucer or a small plate. Leave for a couple of minutes and then push your finger into the jam. If the jam wrinkles then it is ready, if the jam remains runny then return the saucepan back to the heat and boil for a few more minutes before testing again.
7. Remove any scrum from the surface with a spoon.
8. Stir in a knob of butter across the jam surface, this will help to dissolve any remaining scum.
9. Leave the jam to settle for 10-15 minutes
10. Pour the hot jam into warm sterilised jars, seal and label.

Pineapple Jam

Ingredients

- 400g Jam Sugar
- 250ml Water
- 2 Limes, Juice
- 1 Pineapple

Method

1. Grate the flesh of 1 pineapple and place in a large saucepan.
2. Pour in 250ml of water and place over a medium heat. Cook for 30 minutes until the pineapple has softened.
3. Add in 400g of jam sugar to the pineapple and the juice of 2 limes.
4. Cook for 50-60 minutes, until the mixture, becomes thick.
5. Spoon a little of the hot jam onto a chilled saucer or a small plate. Leave for a couple of minutes and then push your finger into the jam. If the jam wrinkles then it is ready, if the jam remains runny then return the saucepan back to the heat and boil for a few more minutes before testing again.
6. Remove any scrum from the surface with a spoon.
7. Leave the jam to settle for 10-15 minutes
8. Pour the hot jam into warm sterilised jars, seal and label.

Peach Jam

Ingredients
- 900g Fresh Peaches
- 900g Golden Granulated Sugar
- 1 Lemon Juice
- Knob of Butter

Method

1. Chop 900g of peaches into chunks, discard the peel and stones.
2. Place the peach chunks in a large saucepan and the juice of 1 lemon.
3. Crush the peach chunks with a masher.
4. Place the saucepan over a medium/high heat and bring to a boil.
5. Reduce the heat and stir in 900g of golden granulated sugar.
6. Stir frequently and bring back to a boil. Boil for a further 15-25 minutes.
7. Spoon a little of the hot jam onto a chilled saucer or a small plate. Leave for a couple of minutes and then push your finger into the jam. If the jam wrinkles then it is ready, if the jam remains runny then return the saucepan back to the heat and boil for a few more minutes before testing again.
8. Remove any scrum from the surface with a spoon.
9. Stir in a knob of butter across the jam surface, this will help to dissolve any remaining scum.
10. Leave the jam to settle for 10-15 minutes
11. Pour the hot jam into warm sterilised jars, seal and label.

Marmalade

Ingredients

- 1.25kg Seville Oranges
- 1.5g Granulated Sugar
- 4 Pints of Water

Method

1. Scrub the oranges well in some fresh clean water.
2. Place the oranges in a large saucepan or a steel pan.
3. Pour in 4 pints of fresh cold water and place the pan over a high heat. Bring to the boil. Reduce the heat and cover the pot with a lid. Simmer for 1 hour until the oranges are soft.
4. Preheat the oven to 140c/gas mark 1.
5. Carefully remove the oranges from the pan with a large spoon and set aside for them to cool.
6. Measure out 3 pints of the orange water and discard any extra, alternatively top up the liquid with fresh water until you have got 3 pints.
7. Place the orange liquid back inside of the pan.
8. Once the oranges have cooled down, cut each of them in half and scoop out the flesh, pith, and pips into a large mixing bowl.
9. Pour the orange pulp into a muslin bag and fasten with a kitchen string. Add the muslin bag to the pan.
10. Chop the orange peels into fine shreds and then add them to the pan.
11. Place the pan over a low heat.
12. Add in 1.5g of granulated sugar and stir until all of the sugar has dissolved.
13. Bring to the boil and cook for 10-15 minutes.
14. Remove any scum from the surface.

15. Spoon a little of the hot marmalade onto a chilled saucer or a small plate. Leave for a couple of minutes and then push your finger into the marmalade. If the marmalade wrinkles, then it is ready if the marmalade remains runny then return the saucepan back to the heat and boil for a few more minutes before testing again.

16. Once the marmalade is ready, remove the pan from the heat.

17. Carefully ladle the hot marmalade into warm sterilised jars. Leave a 1cm space at the top of each jar as the marmalade will continue to thicken up as it cools down. Seal and label.

Popcorn

Toffee Popcorn

Ingredients
- 250g Butter
- 250g Popped Popcorn
- 450g Dark Brown Soft Sugar
- 8 Tablespoons Golden Syrup
- 2 Teaspoons Vanilla Extract
- 1 Teaspoon Salt
- ½ Teaspoon Bicarbonate of Soda

Method

1. Preheat the oven to 120c/ Gas mark 2.
2. Place 250g of popped popcorn in a large mixing bowl.
3. Add 250g of butter to a large saucepan and place over a medium heat. Once all of the butter has melted stir in 450g of dark brown soft sugar, 8 tablespoons of golden syrup and 1 teaspoon of salt.
4. Bring the ingredients to a boil, stirring constantly.
5. Boil for a further 3-4 minutes without stirring.
6. Remove the saucepan from the heat and stir in 2 teaspoons of vanilla extract and ½ teaspoon of bicarbonate of soda.
7. Pour in thin layers over the popcorn, gently stir to ensure all of the popcorn is coated.
8. Divide the popcorn into two large shallow baking dishes and place in the oven.
9. Bake for 50-60 minutes, making sure that you stir the popcorn every 15 minutes.
10. Remove the popcorn from the oven and allow to cool before breaking it up into smaller pieces.
11. Serve.

*Top Tip

This toffee popcorn tastes nice with a side of vanilla ice-cream.

Popcorn Balls

Ingredients
- 400g Caster Sugar
- 250g Popped Popcorn
- 350ml Water
- 175g Golden Syrup
- 10g Butter
- 1 Teaspoon White Vinegar
- 2 Teaspoons of Vanilla Extract
- ½ Teaspoon Salt

Method

1. Place 250g of popped popcorn in a large mixing bowl.
2. Cover a baking tray with a sheet of baking paper.
3. Grease the sides of a large saucepan with some butter.
4. Place 400g of caster sugar, 350ml of water, 175g of golden syrup, 1 teaspoon of white vinegar and ½ teaspoon of salt in the buttered saucepan.
5. Place the saucepan over a medium heat and cook.
6. Stir in 2 teaspoons of vanilla extract. Cook for a further 2-3 minutes.
7. Pour thin layers over the popcorn, gently stir to ensure all of the popcorn is coated.
8. Lightly grease your hands with some butter and carefully shape the popcorn into small balls.
9. Place the balls on the baking paper and allow to cool for at least 60 minutes.
10. Serve.

*Top Tip

You can make the popcorn balls as big or as small as you like.

White Chocolate Popcorn

Ingredients
- 400g Caster Sugar
- 475g white chocolate chips
- 1 tablespoon butter
- 60g Popcorn Kernels
- 2 Tablespoons Coconut Oil

Method

1. Place 2 tablespoons of coconut oil and 60g of popcorn kernels in a large pot and cover with a lid.
2. Place the pot over a medium/high heat.
3. Once the first popcorn pops, remove the pot from the heat and shake the pot well for 20-30 seconds before placing the pot back over the heat.
4. Once most of the popcorn has popped, and it has slowed down, wait 2-3 minutes before removing the pot from the heat.
5. Pour the popcorn out into a large serving bowl.
6. Pour 475g of white chocolate chips into a glass bowl and create a double boiler with a saucepan half full of water.
7. Add 1 tablespoon of butter to the white chocolate chips and melt. Stir frequently for 3-5 minutes, until the chocolate and butter become creamy.
8. Drizzle the melted chocolate over the popcorn. Cover the serving bowl with a lid and shake for a few minutes.
9. Place the popcorn somewhere cool or in the refrigerator to set for approximately 1 hour.
10. Serve.

Coconut Oil Popcorn

Ingredients

- 60g Popcorn Kernels
- 2 Tablespoons Coconut Oil
- Pinch of Sea Salt

Method

1. Place 2 tablespoons of coconut oil and 60g of popcorn kernels in a large pot and cover with a lid.
2. Place the pot over a medium/high heat.
3. Once the first popcorn pops, remove the pot from the heat and shake the pot well for 20-30 seconds before placing the pot back over the heat.
4. Once most of the popcorn has popped, and it has slowed down, wait 2-3 minutes before removing the pot from the heat.
5. Pour the popcorn out into a large serving bowl.
6. Season the popcorn with sea salt to taste.

Salted Popcorn

Ingredients
- 60g Popcorn Kernels
- 3 Tablespoons Peanut Oil
- 2 Tablespoons Butter
- A Pinch of Sea Salt

Method

1. Place 3 tablespoons of peanut oil and 60g of popcorn kernels in a large pot.
2. Sprinkle some sea salt on the kernels; you can add as much or as little salt as you like.
3. Add in 2 tablespoons of butter and cover the pot with a lid.
4. Place the pot over a medium/high heat.
5. Once the first popcorn pops, remove the pot from the heat and shake the pot well for 20-30 seconds before placing the pot back over the heat.
6. Once most of the popcorn has popped, and it has slowed down, wait 2-3 minutes before removing the pot from the heat.
7. Pour the popcorn out into a large serving bowl.
8. Season the popcorn with a pinch of sea salt to taste.
9. Serve.

Sweet Popcorn

Ingredients

- 60g Popcorn Kernels
- 4 Tablespoons Butter
- 3 Tablespoons Icing Sugar
- 1 Tablespoon Coconut Oil

Method

1. Place 4 tablespoons of butter in a large pan and place over a medium/high heat until all of the butter has melted.
2. Mix in 3 tablespoons of icing sugar. Stir the ingredients together until all of the icing sugar has fully dissolved.
3. Add 1 tablespoon of coconut oil to the pan.
4. Add 60g of popcorn kernels to the ingredients. Swirl the pan so that the oil just about covers the kernels.
5. Place a lid over the pot.
6. Increase the heat to high.
7. Once the first popcorn pops, remove the pot from the heat and shake the pot well for 20-30 seconds before placing the pot back over the heat. You may need to shake the pop more frequently during cooking as the added icing sugar can cause the kernels to stick and burn to pot.
8. Once most of the popcorn has popped and it has slowed down, wait 2-3 minutes before removing the pot from the heat.
9. Pour the popcorn out into a large serving bowl.
10. Serve.

Lemon Popcorn

Ingredients
- 60g Popcorn Kernels
- 2 Tablespoons of coconut/ peanut oil
- 2 Tablespoons of Lemon Juice
- 2 Tablespoons of Butter
- Salt to Taste (Optional)

Method

1. Place 2 tablespoons of coconut oil and 60g of popcorn kernels in a large pot and cover with a lid.
2. Place the pot over a medium/high heat.
3. Once the first popcorn pops, remove the pot from the heat and shake the pot well for 20-30 seconds before placing the pot back over the heat.
4. Once most of the popcorn has popped, and it has slowed, down wait 2-3 minutes before removing the pot from the heat.
5. Pour the popcorn out into a large serving bowl.
6. Add 2 tablespoons of butter to a small saucepan and 2 tablespoons of lemon juice. Place the saucepan over a medium heat and stir the ingredients together until all of the butter has melted.
7. Drizzle the melted lemon butter over the popcorn. Cover the serving bowl with a lid and shake for a few minutes.
8. Place the popcorn somewhere cool or in the refrigerator to set for approximately 1 hour.
9. To Season you can add a pinch of sea salt to taste.
10. Serve.

Sauces & Dips

Mayonnaise

Ingredients

- 2 Egg Yolks
- 1 Egg
- ½ Teaspoon Caster Sugar
- ½ Lemon
- 400ml Vegetable Oil
- 1 Tablespoon of Mustard
- Pinch of Salt
- Pinch of Ground Black Pepper

Method

1. Crack 1 egg into a mixing bowl and add in 2 egg yolks, whisk together.
2. Add in ½ teaspoon of caster sugar and 1 tablespoon of mustard to the eggs.
3. Juice ½ a lemon and pour into the mixing bowl. Whisk the ingredients together for 2-3 minutes, alternatively, place the ingredients in a blender or a food processor and blend for 15-20 seconds until all of the ingredients are well combined.
4. Once the egg mixture has become thick and glossy, gradually mix in 400ml of vegetable oil. If you are using a blender add the vegetable oil and blend for a further 20-30 seconds.
5. Add a pinch of salt and a pinch of ground black pepper.
6. Serve.

*Top Tip

You can season the mayonnaise to suit your personal taste by adding more or less salt and ground black pepper.

Tomato Sauce

Ingredients
- 2.5kg Tinned Chopped Tomatoes
- 100g Tomato Puree
- 70g Apple Cider Vinegar or Distilled White Vinegar
- 3 Onions
- 6 Tablespoons of Honey
- 1/8 Teaspoon Celery Salt
- 2 Carrots
- 4 Cloves of Garlic
- 1/8 Teaspoon Mustard Powder
- ¼ Teaspoon Ground Black Pepper
- 1 Teaspoon Salt
- 2 Tablespoons of Rapeseed Oil

Method

1. Peel and chop 3 onions, 4 cloves of garlic and 2 carrots up into small pieces.
2. Add 2 tablespoons of rapeseed oil to a saucepan and place over a medium heat.
3. Add the chopped vegetables to the saucepan and cook uncovered for 15 minutes.
4. Add in 100g of tomato puree to the vegetables and cook for a further 1-2 minutes.
5. Add 6 tablespoons of honey and stir the ingredients.
6. Pour in 70g of apple cider or distilled white vinegar.
7. Stir in 2.5kg of tinned chopped tomatoes.
8. Add ¼ teaspoon of ground black pepper, 1/8 teaspoon of mustard powder, 1/8 teaspoon of celery salt and 1 teaspoon of salt to the tomato sauce and stir well.

9.   Bring the sauce to a boil and simmer for 30-40 minutes on a low heat.
10. Remove the tomato sauce from the heat and purée in a blender or with an immersion blender.
11. Store in a clean glass jar and serve cold.

*Top Tip

This tomato sauce goes well with fish cakes, fish fingers, homemade chips, and breaded chicken. The tomato sauce can also be frozen

Hummus

Ingredients
- 200g Tinned Chickpeas
- 3 Tablespoons of Lemon Juice
- 3 Cloves of Garlic
- 1 Teaspoon Ground Cumin
- 100ml Tahini
- 4 Tablespoons of Water
- 1 Teaspoon Paprika
- ½ Teaspoon Salt
- 2 Tablespoons of Extra Virgin Olive Oil

Method

1. Drain 200g of tinned chickpeas and rinse in cold fresh water. Once drained place the chickpeas in a medium sized bowl. Take a small handful of chickpeas and leave to one side for serving.
2. Peel and chop 3 cloves of garlic up into small pieces.
3. Place the chickpeas, garlic, 3 tablespoons of lemon juice, 1 teaspoon of ground cumin, ½ teaspoon of salt, 100ml of tahini and 4 tablespoons of water in a blender or a food processor and blend until a creamy puree is formed.
4. Pour the hummus out onto a plate or a bowl and smooth out with the back of a spoon.
5. Drizzle 2 tablespoons of extra virgin olive oil over the hummus.
6. Scatter a handful of the reserved chickpeas over the hummus and sprinkle the top with 1 teaspoon of paprika.

*Top Tip

You can add more lemon juice, garlic, cumin, paprika or salt to suit your personal taste.

Guacamole

Ingredients

- 3 Avocados
- 1 Lime
- 75g Onion
- 2 Tomatoes
- 1 Teaspoon of Minced Garlic
- ½ Teaspoon Cayenne Pepper
- 3 Tablespoons Chopped Fresh Cilantro
- 1 Teaspoon of Salt

Method

1. Peel and pit 3 avocados and place them in a medium sized bowl.
2. Juice 1 Lime and add 1 teaspoon of salt to the avocados before mashing all of the ingredients together.
3. Peel and chop 75g of onion into small pieces. Mix the onion in with the avocado.
4. Chop 2 tomatoes up into small pieces and add to the bowl along with 3 tablespoons of fresh chopped cilantro.
5. Stir in ½ teaspoon of cayenne pepper and 1 teaspoon of minced garlic.
6. Mix the ingredients together well and then refrigerate for 1/2 hours to allow the flavors to immerse.
7. Serve.

Garlic & Chive Dip

Ingredients

- 3 Cloves of Garlic
- 100ml Soured Cream
- 100ml crème Fraiche
- 2 Tablespoons of Chopped Fresh Chives
- 2 Tablespoons Lemon Juice
- ½ Teaspoon Ground Black Pepper

Method

1. Peel and chop 3 cloves of garlic into small segments and then crush the garlic with a pestle and mortar, alternatively, you can use a garlic press.
2. Place the garlic in a blender or in a food processor along with 100ml of soured cream, 100ml of crème Fraiche, 2 tablespoons of fresh chopped chives and blend for 1-2 minutes, or until the ingredients are smooth.
3. Stir in 2 tablespoons of lemon juice and ½ teaspoon of ground black pepper. Blend for a further 1-2 minutes.
4. Pour the garlic and chive dip into a small condiment bowl and serve.

*Top Tip

You can add more or less garlic and chives to suit your personal taste.

Avocado & Mango Salsa

Ingredients

- 1 Avocado
- 1 Mango
- 1 Lime
- 1 Red Onion
- 1 Scotch Bonnet Chili
- 1 Tablespoon Fresh Chopped Coriander
- Pinch of Salt
- Pinch of Ground Black Pepper

Method

1. Peel and pit 1 avocado and then chop into really small pieces. Place the avocado in a serving bowl.
2. Peel and deseed 1 whole mango and chop into tiny pieces. Add the mango to the avocado in the serving bowl.
3. Peel and chop 1 red onion into small pieces and 1 Scotch bonnet chili. Stir the red onion and scotch bonnet chili pieces into the serving bowl.
4. Add 1 tablespoon of finely chopped fresh coriander, a pinch of salt and pinch of ground black pepper and mix the ingredients together.
5. Serve immediately or refrigerate for one hour.

Salsa

Ingredients
- ½ Cucumber
- 4 Tomatoes
- 4 Spring Onions
- 2 Mild Chilies
- 10ml Extra Virgin Olive Oil
- ½ Lemon
- Handful of Mint Leaves
- Handful of Parsley
- 1 Tablespoon of Water
- Pinch of Salt

Method

1. Chop ½ a cucumber and 4 tomatoes up into small chunks and place in a mixing bowl.
2. Cut 4 spring onions up into small pieces and 2 mild chilies and add them to the mixing bowl.
3. Finely chop 1 handful of mint leaves and 1 handful of parsley, add the herbs to the mixing bowl and stir together.
4. Juice ½ of a lemon and pour the liquid into a small bowl.
5. Add 10ml extra virgin olive oil to the lemon juice.
6. Pour the ingredients out into the small bowl and add in a pinch of salt. Stir the ingredients together.
7. Cover and refrigerate or serve immediately.

Chutney

Ingredients

- 1kg Apples
- 500g Onions
- 2 Garlic Cloves
- ¼ Piece of Fresh Root Ginger
- 250g Brown Sugar
- 85g Sultanas
- 500ml Distilled Malt Vinegar
- ¼ Teaspoon Dried Chili Flakes
- ½ Teaspoon Salt

Method

1. Peel and chop 1kg of apples into small pieces, discard the cores and skin. Place the apple chunks in a large saucepan.
2. Peel and chop 500g of onions into small pieces and add to the apple chunks.
3. Finely chop 2 cloves of garlic and ¼ pieces of fresh root ginger and add to the saucepan.
4. Add 250g brown sugar, ½ teaspoon of salt and ¼ teaspoon of dried chili flakes to the ingredients.
5. Place the saucepan over a medium heat and stir.
6. Gradually stir in 500ml of distilled malt vinegar.
7. Once all of the brown sugar has dissolved, bring to the boil and then simmer on a low heat for approximately 55-60 minutes, stirring the ingredients occasionally.
8. When the chutney has thickened stir more often to ensure that the sugar does not burn and stick to the bottom of the saucepan.
9. Carefully spoon the chutney into some clean glass jars. Store the jars in a cool, dark place for a month before eating.

Ice Teas

Ice Tea

Ingredients
- 4 Tea Bags
- 550ml Hot Water
- 550ml Cold Water
- 85g Caster Sugar

Method

1. Fill a pitcher with 550ml hot water and 550ml cold water.
2. Add in 4 tea bags to the water.
3. Cover the pitcher and steep for 8-12 hours in the refrigerator.
4. Serve.

*Top Tip

Add in ice cubes before serving the ice tea. You can also substitute the sugar for honey and add more or less to suit your personal taste.

Blueberry Ice Tea

Ingredients

- 250g Blueberries
- 550ml Water
- 550ml Brewed Tea
- 85g Caster Sugar
- 60ml Lemon Juice

Method

1. Place 250g of blueberries in a large saucepan and add in 60ml of lemon juice. Place the saucepan over a medium heat and bring to a boil. Cook for a further 5 minutes, stirring occasionally.
2. Remove the saucepan from the heat and strain the liquid into a large mixing bowl. Use the back of a spoon to squeeze any juice out of the fruit.
3. Stir in 85g of caster sugar and 550ml of brewed tea.
4. Pour the liquid out into a pitcher and cover. Place the pitcher in the refrigerator and leave to chill for at least 1 hour.
5. Serve.

*Top Tip

Add in some ice cubes before serving the ice tea. You can also substitute the sugar for honey and add more or less to suit your personal taste.

Raspberry Ice Tea

Ingredients
- 550ml Water
- 550ml Brewed Tea
- 250g Raspberries
- 85g Caster Sugar

Method

1. Place 250g of raspberries in a large saucepan and 550ml of fresh cold water. Place the saucepan over a medium heat and bring to a boil. Cook for a further five minutes, stirring occasionally.
2. Remove the saucepan from the heat and strain the liquid into a large mixing bowl. Use the back of a spoon to squeeze any juice out of the fruit.
3. Stir in 85g of caster sugar and 550ml of brewed tea.
4. Pour the liquid out into a pitcher and cover. Place the pitcher in the refrigerator and leave to chill for at least 1 hour.
5. Serve.

*Top Tip

Add in some ice cubes before serving the ice tea. You can also substitute the sugar for honey and add more or less to suit your personal taste.

Orange Ice Tea

Ingredients

- 550ml Brewed Tea
- 85g Caster Sugar
- 2 Blood Orange
- 1 Teaspoon Vanilla
- Sprinkle of Cinnamon

Method

1. Chop 2 blood oranges into thin slices and place in the bottom of a pitcher.
2. Add 1 teaspoon of vanilla and a sprinkle of cinnamon to the orange slices.
3. Add 85g of caster sugar to the pitcher.
4. Pour in 550ml of brewed tea into the pitcher whilst it is still hot to ensure that the sugar dissolves.
5. Stir well.
6. Place the pitcher in the refrigerator and leave to chill for at least 1 hour.
7. Serve.

*Top Tip

Add in some ice cubes before serving the ice tea. You can also substitute the sugar for honey and add more or less to suit your personal taste.

Strawberry Ice Tea

Ingredients

- 550ml Brewed Tea
- 150ml Water
- 450g Strawberries
- 85g Caster Sugar

Method

1. Remove the leafs from 450g of strawberries and cut into halves.
2. Place 450g of strawberries in a large saucepan along with 150ml of cold fresh water and 85g of caster sugar. Place the saucepan over a medium heat and bring to a boil. Simmer for a further fifteen minutes, stirring occasionally.
3. Remove the saucepan from the heat and strain the liquid into a large mixing bowl. Use the back of a spoon to squeeze any juice out of the fruit.
4. Stir in 550ml of brewed tea.
5. Pour the liquid out into a pitcher and cover. Place the pitcher in the refrigerator and leave to chill for at least 1 hour.
6. Serve.

*Top Tip

Add in some ice cubes before serving the ice tea. You can also substitute the sugar for honey and add more or less to suit your personal taste.

Peach Ice Tea

Ingredients
- 160ml Peach Nectar
- 550ml Brewed Tea
- 85g Caster Sugar

Method

1. Pour 160ml of peach nectar into a pitcher.
2. Add in 550ml of brewed tea and 85g of caster sugar to the pitcher.
3. Stir the ingredients together until all of the sugar has fully dissolved.
4. Cover and place the pitcher in the refrigerator and leave to chill for at least 1 hour.
5. Serve.

*Top Tip

Add in some ice cubes before serving the ice tea. You can also substitute the sugar for honey and add more or less to suit your personal taste.

Lime Mint Ice Tea

Ingredients
- 550ml Brewed Tea
- 85g Caster Sugar
- Juice of 3 Limes
- A Handful of Fresh Mint Leaves

Method

1. Pour 550ml of brewed tea into a pitcher.
2. Stir in 85g of caster sugar and the juice from 3 limes. Mix the ingredients together until all of the sugar has dissolved.
3. Add a handful of fresh mint leaves to the ice tea and stir.
4. Cover and place the pitcher in the refrigerator and leave to chill for at least 1 hour.
5. Serve.

*Top Tip

Add in some ice cubes before serving the ice tea. You can also substitute the sugar for honey and add more or less to suit your personal taste.

Citrus Ice Tea

Ingredients

- 550ml Water
- 2 Regular Teabags
- 85g Caster Sugar
- Juice of 2 Lemons
- 1 Cinnamon Stick
- 1 Orange
- 1 Lemon
- 1 Lime
- ½ Cucumber

Method

1. Fill a large saucepan with 550ml of fresh cold water.
2. Add in 1 cinnamon stick and 85g of sugar to the saucepan and place over a medium/high heat. Stir the ingredients together until all of the sugar has dissolved. Bring the water to the boil.
3. Remove the saucepan from the heat.
4. Hang 2 regular tea bags in the boiling water. Cover the saucepan and leave to rest for at least 50-60 minutes.
5. Remove the cinnamon stick from the saucepan and pour the tea into a pitcher.
6. Stir in the juice of 2 lemons.
7. Chop 1 orange, 1 lemon, 1 lime and ½ cucumber up into small slices or into small chunks and add to the tea.
8. Cover and place the pitcher in the refrigerator and leave to chill for at least 1 hour.
9. Serve.

*Top Tip

Add in some ice cubes before serving the ice tea. You can also substitute the sugar for honey and add more or less to suit your personal taste.

Infusion Waters

Lemon Water

Ingredients
- 1 Jug of Fresh Cold Water
- 1-2 Lemons
- 6 Ice Cubes

Method

1. Cut 1-2 lemons up into thin slices and add them to the jug of fresh cold water.
2. Add 6 ice cubes into the jug of water.
3. Place the jug in the refrigerator for 2-4 hours to allow the lemons to infuse.
4. Stir well & serve.

*Top Tip

You can keep the infused water refrigerated for up to 2 days.

Blueberry Lime Water

Ingredients

- 1 Jug of Sparkling or Still Water
- 50g Fresh Blueberries
- 1½ Limes
- 6 Ice Cubes

Method

1. Add 50g of fresh blueberries to 1 jug of sparkling or still water.
2. Cut 1½ limes up into thin slices and place in the jug of water.
3. Add 6 ice cubes to the jug of water.
4. Place the jug in the refrigerator for 2-4 hours to allow the fruit to infuse.
5. Stir well & serve.

*Top Tip

You can keep the infused water refrigerated for up to 2 days.

Lemon Cucumber Water

Ingredients

- 1 Jug of Sparkling or Still Water
- 1 Lemon
- ½ Cucumber
- 6 Ice Cubes

Method

1. Chop 1 lemon up into thin slices and add to the jug of water.
2. Chop ½ cucumber up into thin slices and add to the jug of water.
3. Add 6 ice cubes to the fruit water.
4. Place the jug in the refrigerator for 2-4 hours to allow the fruit to infuse.
5. Stir well & serve.

*Top Tip

You can keep the infused water refrigerated for up to 2 days.

Blueberry, Apple & Raspberry Water

Ingredients
- 1 Jug of Sparkling or Still Water
- 40g Fresh Blueberries
- 40g Fresh Raspberries
- 2 Red Apples
- 6 Ice Cubes

Method

1. Chop 2 red apples up into thin wedges and add to the jug of water.
2. Add 40g of fresh blueberries and 40g of fresh raspberries to the jug of water.
3. Add 6 ice cubes to the fruit water.
4. Place the jug in the refrigerator for 2-4 hours to allow the fruit to infuse.
5. Stir well & serve.

*Top Tip

You can keep the infused water refrigerated for up to 2 days.

Blueberry Lavender Water

Ingredients

- 1 Jug of Sparkling or Still Water
- 220g Fresh Blueberries
- 1 Handful of Lavender Flowers
- 6 Ice Cubes

Method

1. Add 220g of fresh blueberries to the jug of water.
2. Add 1 handful of lavender flowers to the jug of water.
3. Add 6 ice cubes to the fruit water.
4. Place the jug in the refrigerator for 2-4 hours to allow the fruit to infuse.
5. Stir well & serve.

*Top Tip

You can keep the infused water refrigerated for up to 2 days.

Apple, Ginger & Lemongrass Water

Ingredients

- 1 Jug of Sparkling or Still Water
- 3 Red Apples
- 2 Lemongrass Sticks
- 1 Inch Ginger Root
- 6 Ice Cubes

Method

1. Chop 3 red apples up into small wedge chunks and add to the jug of water.
2. Peel and chop 1 inch of ginger root up into small pieces and add to the water.
3. Add 2 lemongrass sticks to the jug of water.
4. Add 6 ice cubes to the fruit water.
5. Place the jug in the refrigerator for 2-4 hours to allow the fruit to infuse.
6. Stir well & serve.

*Top Tip

You can keep the infused water refrigerated for up to 2 days. You can also grate the ginger root for a more intense flavour.

Watermelon Mint Water

Ingredients

- ☐1 Jug of Sparkling or Still Water
- 180g Watermelon
- 1 Handful of Fresh Mint Leaves
- 6 Ice Cubes

Method

1. Chop 180g of watermelon up into small cubes and add to the jug of water.
2. Add 1 handful of fresh mint leaves to the jug of water.
3. Add 6 ice cubes to the fruit water.
4. Place the jug in the refrigerator for 2-4 hours to allow the fruit to infuse.
5. Stir well & serve.

*Top Tip

You can keep the infused water refrigerated for up to 2 days.

Orange Kiwi Water

Ingredients

- 1 Jug of Sparkling or Still Water
- 1 Orange
- 2 Kiwis
- 6 Ice Cubes

Method

1. Chop 1 orange up into thin slices and add to the jug of water.
2. Peel and chop 2 kiwis up into thin slices and add to the jug of water.
3. Add 6 ice cubes to the fruit water.
4. Place the jug in the refrigerator for 2-4 hours to allow the fruit to infuse.
5. Stir well & serve.

*Top Tip

You can keep the infused water refrigerated for up to 2 days.

Raspberry Mint Water

Ingredients

- 1 Jug of Sparkling or Still Water
- 65g Fresh Raspberries
- Handful of Fresh Mint
- 6 Ice Cubes

Method

1. Add 65g of fresh raspberries to 1 jug of sparkling or still water.
2. Add in a handful of fresh mint to the water and stir.
3. Add 6 ice cubes into the jug of water.
4. Place the jug in the refrigerator for 2-4 hours to allow the fruit to infuse.
5. Stir well & serve.

*Top Tip

You can keep the infused water refrigerated for up to 2 days.

Strawberry Basil Water

Ingredients

- 1 Jug of Sparkling or Still Water
- 90g Fresh Strawberries
- Handful of Fresh Basil
- 6 Ice Cubes

Method

1. Chop 90g of fresh strawberries up into thin slices and add to 1 jug of sparkling or still water.
2. Add in a handful of fresh basil to the water and stir.
3. Add 6 ice cubes into the jug of water.
4. Place the jug in the refrigerator for 2-4 hours to allow the fruit to infuse.
5. Stir well & serve.

*Top Tip

You can keep the infused water refrigerated for up to 2 days.

Rose Lemon & Strawberry Water

Ingredients

- 1 Jug of Sparkling or Still Water
- 85g Fresh Strawberries
- 1 Lemon
- Handful of Fresh Rose Petals (Pesticide Free)
- 6 Ice Cubes

Method

1. Chop 85g of fresh strawberries in half and add to the jug of sparkling or still water.
2. Chop 1 lemon up into thin slices and add to the jug of water.
3. Add a handful of fresh rose petals into the fruit water.
4. Add 6 ice cubes into the jug of water.
5. Place the jug in the refrigerator for 2-4 hours to allow the fruit to infuse.
6. Stir well & serve.

*Top Tip

You can keep the infused water refrigerated for up to 2 days.

Mango, Cucumber & Ginger Water

Ingredients

- 1 Jug of Sparkling or Still Water
- 90g Fresh Mango
- ½ Cucumber
- 1 Inch Ginger Root
- 6 Ice Cubes

Method

1. Peel and chop 90g of fresh mango up into small chunks and add to the jug of sparkling or still water.
2. Chop ½ cucumber up into small thin slices and place them in the jug of water.
3. Peel and chop 1 inch of ginger root and add to the water.
4. Add in 6 ice cubes to the jug of water.
5. Place the jug in the refrigerator for 2-4 hours to allow the fruit to infuse.
6. Stir well & serve.

*Top Tip

You can keep the infused water refrigerated for up to 2 days. You can also grate the ginger root for a more intense flavour.

Grape, Raspberry & Cucumber Water

Ingredients

- 1 Jug of Sparkling or Still Water
- 40g Fresh Grapes
- 40g Fresh Raspberry
- ½ Cucumber
- 6 Ice Cubes

Method

1. Add 40g of fresh grapes and 40g of fresh raspberries to the jug of sparkling or still water.
2. Chop ½ cucumber up into small thin slices and add to the jug of water.
3. Add in 6 ice cubes to the jug of water.
4. Place the jug in the refrigerator for 2-4 hours to allow the fruit to infuse.
5. Stir well & serve.

*Top Tip

You can keep the infused water refrigerated for up to 2 days.

Pineapple, Lemon & Pomegranate Water

Ingredients
- 1 Jug of Sparkling or Still Water
- 80g Fresh Pineapple
- 1 Lemon
- 2 Fresh Pomegranates
- 6 Ice Cubes

Method

1. Chop 80g of fresh pineapple up into small square chunks and add to the jug of sparkling or still water.
2. Chop 1 lemon up into thin slices and add to the jug of water.
3. Deseed 2 fresh pomegranates and add to the fruit water.
4. Add in 6 ice cubes to the jug of water.
5. Place the jug in the refrigerator for 2-4 hours to allow the fruit to infuse.
6. Stir well & serve.

*Top Tip

You can keep the infused water refrigerated for up to 2 days.

Orange, Strawberry & Cranberry Water

Ingredients
- 1 Jug of Sparkling or Still Water
- 1 Blood Orange
- 1 Lemon
- 75g Fresh Strawberries
- A Handful of Fresh Cranberries
- 6 Ice Cubes

Method

1. Chop 1 blood orange and 1 lemon up into thin slices and add to the jug of sparkling or still water.
2. Chop 75g of fresh strawberries in half and place them in the jug of water.
3. Add a handful of fresh cranberries to the fruit water.
4. Add in 6 ice cubes to the jug of water.
5. Place the jug in the refrigerator for 2-4 hours to allow the fruit to infuse.
6. Stir well & serve.

*Top Tip

You can keep the infused water refrigerated for up to 2 days.

Drinks

Real Strawberry Milkshake

Ingredients
- 200g Strawberries
- 120ml Whole Milk
- 2 Teaspoons Sugar
- 1 Teaspoon Vanilla Extract
- 4 Scoops of Vanilla Ice Cream

Method

1. Place 200g of fresh or frozen strawberries in a mixing bowl.
2. Add in 2 teaspoons of sugar and 1 teaspoon of vanilla extract to the strawberries. Mix the ingredients together and set aside for 15-20 minutes.
3. Place the strawberry mixture into a blender and add in 4 scoops of vanilla ice cream and 120ml of milk.
4. Blitz the blender for 1-2 minutes, or until the mixture is smooth.
5. Pour the milkshake out into a tall highball glass.
6. The drink is ready to serve.

Real Raspberry Milkshake

Ingredients
- 200g Raspberries
- 120ml Whole Milk
- 2 Teaspoons Sugar
- 1 Teaspoon Vanilla Extract
- 4 Scoops of Vanilla Ice Cream

Method

1. Place 200g of fresh or frozen raspberries in a mixing bowl.
2. Add 2 teaspoons of sugar and 1 teaspoon of vanilla extract to the raspberries. Mix the ingredients together and set aside for 15-20 minutes.
3. Place the raspberry mixture into a blender and add in 4 scoops of vanilla ice cream and 120ml of milk.
4. Blitz the blender for 1-2 minutes, or until the mixture is smooth.
5. Pour the milkshake out into a tall highball glass.
6. The drink is ready to serve.

Real Banana Milkshake

Ingredients
- 250g Bananas
- 120ml Whole Milk
- 2 Teaspoons Sugar
- 1 Teaspoon Vanilla Extract
- 4 Scoops of Vanilla Ice Cream

Method

1. Place 200g of fresh or frozen bananas in a mixing bowl.
2. Add in 2 teaspoons of sugar and 1 teaspoon of vanilla extract to the bananas. Mix the ingredients together and set aside for 15-20 minutes.
3. Place the banana mixture into a blender and add in 4 scoops of vanilla ice cream and 120ml of milk.
4. Blitz the blender for 1-2 minutes, or until the mixture is smooth.
5. Pour the milkshake out into a tall highball glass.
6. The drink is ready to serve.

Lemonade

Ingredients

- 4 Lemons
- 160g Caster Sugar
- 1 Liter Cold Water
- Lemon/Lime Slices
- Ice Cubes

Method

1. Roughly peel and chop 4 lemons.
2. Place the lemon pieces in a blender or in a food processor along with 160g of caster sugar and half of the cold water.
3. Blitz the blender for 1-2 minutes.
4. Place a sieve over a large bowl and pour the lemonade out into it. Use the back of a spoon to press any juicy bits.
5. Add the other half of the cold water to the lemonade.
6. Place the lemonade in a large jug or carefully pour it out into a sterilised glass bottle.
7. Garnish with some slices of lemon or lime.
8. Serve with ice cubes.

*Top Tip

The lemonade can be stored in the refrigerator for up to one week.

Pink Lemonade

Ingredients
- 300g Caster Sugar
- 350ml Cold Water
- 350g Raspberries
- 3 Lemons
- A Handful of Fresh Mint
- Ice Cubes

Method

1. Place 350g of raspberries in a large saucepan and pour over 350ml of cold water.
2. Roughly peel and chop 3 lemons and add them to the saucepan along with 300g of caster sugar.
3. Place the saucepan on a medium/high heat and bring to a boil. Occasionally stir the ingredients.
4. Allow the liquid to cool.
5. Place a sieve over a large bowl and pour the lemonade out into it. Use the back of a spoon to press any juicy bits.
6. Pour the lemonade out into a large jug or carefully pour it out into a sterilised glass bottle.
7. Top up the syrup with cold still water or sparkling water.
8. Place the lemonade in the fridge for at least 1-2 hours.
9. Garnish with a handful of fresh mint.
10. Serve with ice cubes.

*Top Tip

The lemonade can be stored in the refrigerator for up to one week.

Watermelon & Strawberry Lemonade

Ingredients
- 1.1kg Watermelon
- 465ml Cold Water
- 200g Caster Sugar
- 150g Strawberries
- 120ml Lemon Juice, Fresh

Method

1. Deseed and cube 1.1kg of fresh watermelon.
2. Slice 150g of strawberries in half.
3. Place the cubed watermelon and strawberries in a blender or in a food processor along with 120ml of lemon juice and 200g of caster sugar.
4. Add 465ml of cold water to the blender.
5. Blitz the blender for 1-2 minutes, or until the mixture is smooth.
6. Pour the lemonade out into a large jug or carefully pour it out into a sterilised glass bottle.
7. Place the lemonade in the fridge for at least 1-2 hours.
8. Serve with ice cubes.

*Top Tip

The lemonade can be stored in the refrigerator for up to one week.

Orange Lemonade

Ingredients

- 70g Caster Sugar
- 565ml Cold Water
- 120ml Orange Juice, Fresh
- 120ml Lemon Juice, Fresh
- 2 Tablespoons Grated Lemon Peel
- 2 Tablespoons Grated Orange Peel

Method

1. Place 70g of caster sugar in a large saucepan and pour in half of the cold water.
2. Place the saucepan over a medium/high heat and cook until all of the sugar has dissolved.
3. Remove the saucepan from the heat and leave the liquid to cool slightly.
4. Stir in 2 tablespoons of grated lemon peel and 2 tablespoons of grated orange peel.
5. Pour in 120ml of fresh orange juice and 120ml of fresh lemon juice.
6. Gently stir the ingredients
7. Cover the saucepan and set aside for at least 1 hour.
8. Strain the syrup and add the remaining cold water.
9. Place the lemonade in a large jug or carefully pour it out into a sterilised glass bottle.
10. Place the lemonade in the fridge for at least 1-2 hours.
11. Serve with ice cubes.

*Top Tip

The lemonade can be stored in the refrigerator for up to one week.

Watermelon Slush

Ingredients

- 1.2kg Watermelon
- Lime Juice, Fresh
- 2 Tablespoons Caster Sugar
- 12-15 Ice Cubes

Method

1. Deseed and cube 1.1kg of fresh watermelon.
2. Place the watermelon in a blender along with the juice of 1 lime, 2 tablespoons of caster sugar and 12-15 ice cubes.
3. Blitz the blender for 1-2 minutes.
4. Pour the watermelon slush out into a tall highball glass.
5. The drink is ready to serve.

Banana Berry Slush

Ingredients
- 2 Ripe Bananas
- 220g Frozen Berries (Strawberries, Raspberries, Cranberries, Blackberries)
- 10-12 Ice Cubes

Method

1. Slice 2 ripe bananas into small chunks and place them in a blender.
2. Add 220g of frozen berries to the blender and 10-12 ice cubes.
3. Blitz the blender for 1-2 minutes.
4. Pour the slush out into a tall highball glass
5. The drink is ready to serve.

Orange Slush

Ingredients
- 120ml Orange Juice
- 60ml Milk
- 2 Tablespoons Caster Sugar
- 12-15 Ice Cubes

Method

1. Pour 120ml of orange juice and 60ml of milk into a blender and add 2 tablespoons of caster sugar.
2. Add 12-15 ice cubes to the blender.
3. Blitz the blender for 1-2 minutes or until smooth.
4. Pour the orange slush out into a tall highball glass
5. The drink is ready to serve.

Blueberry Cream Slush

Ingredients

- 140g Frozen Blueberries
- 140g Frozen Strawberries
- 140g Vanilla Yogurt
- 60ml Pineapple Juice
- 60ml Orange Juice
- 2 Teaspoons Caster Sugar
- 6-8 Ice Cubes

Method

1. Place 140g of frozen blueberries and 140g of frozen strawberries in a blender.
2. Add 140g of vanilla yogurt to the blender and 2 teaspoons of caster sugar.
3. Blitz the blender for 1-2 minutes.
4. Pour in 60ml of pineapple juice and 60ml of orange juice.
5. Add 6-8 ice cubes to the blender and blend for a further 1-2 minutes.
6. Pour the slush out into a tall highball glass.
7. The drink is ready to serve.

Homemade Cordial

Elderflower

Ingredients

- 15-20 Heads of Elderflower

- 500g Caster Sugar

- 4 Tablespoons Clear Honey

- 2 Lemons, Unwaxed

- 1 Liter Cold Water

Method

1. Wash 15-20 heads of elderflower extremely well, making sure that there are no bugs on them.
2. Place 500g of caster sugar in a large saucepan and add 4 tablespoons of clear honey.
3. Pour in 1 liter of cold water over the sugar.
4. Place the saucepan over a medium/high heat and gently bring to a boil.
5. Boil until all of the sugar has dissolved, gently stirring the liquid from time to time.
6. Remove the saucepan from the heat.
7. Finely grate in the zest of 2 unwaxed lemons.
8. Place 15-20 heads of elderflower in upside down. Ensure that the elderflower heads are completely submerged in the liquid.
9. Squeeze the juice from 1 of the unwaxed lemons into the saucepan.
10. Chop the other lemon into thin slices and add it to the saucepan.

11. Cover the saucepan with a lid and set aside for at least 24 hours to allow the ingredients to infuse.
12. Line a fine sieve with a muslin. Place the sieve over a large bowl.
13. Strain the cordial by pouring it out into the sieve.
14. Transfer the cordial into sterilised bottles or jars and seal.
15. Serve diluted with water.

*Top Tip

You can substitute the water and dilute the elderflower cordial with soda or prosecco. Once you have opened the cordial, store in the refrigerator.

Raspberry

Ingredients

- 150ml Apple Juice

- 500g Raspberries

- 500g Caster Sugar

- 300ml Cold Water

- 3 Tablespoons Red Wine Vinegar

Method

1. Place 500g of raspberries in a large saucepan.
2. Add 3 tablespoons of red wine vinegar to the raspberries and 500g of caster sugar.
3. Place the saucepan over a low heat and mash the raspberries until they turn smooth and syrupy, for approximately 10-12 minutes.
4. Place a sieve over a clean saucepan and pour the ingredients through the sieve.
5. Place the raspberry seeds from the sieve into a bowl and stir in 300ml of cold water.
6. Sieve again to remove the last bit of pulp from the seeds.
7. Pour the liquid into the saucepan with the sieved pulp and stir well.
8. Place the saucepan over a medium heat and boil for 1-2 minutes.
9. Transfer the cordial into sterilised bottles or jars and seal.
10. Serve diluted with water.

*Top Tip

You can substitute the water and dilute the raspberry cordial with soda or prosecco. Once you have opened the cordial, store in the refrigerator.

Strawberry

Ingredients
- 300g Strawberries, Ripe
- 375g Granulated Sugar
- 1.5 Liters of Cold Water

Method

1. Place 375g of granulated sugar in a large saucepan.
2. Pour in 1.5 liters of cold water over the sugar and place the saucepan over a low heat.
3. Once the sugar has dissolved, increase the heat to medium/high and bring to a boil.
4. Chop 300g of strawberries in half and add to the saucepan.
5. Cover the saucepan with a lid and remove from the heat.
6. Leave the saucepan to one side for at least 1 hour to allow the ingredients to infuse.
7. Line a fine sieve with a muslin. Place the sieve over a large bowl.
8. Strain the cordial by pouring it into the sieve. Leave the pulp to drip until all of the liquid has been collected.
9. Transfer the cordial into sterilised bottles or jars and seal.
10. Chill in the refrigerator.
11. Serve diluted with water.

*Top Tip

You can substitute the water and dilute the strawberry cordial with soda or prosecco. Once you have opened the cordial, store in the refrigerator.

Lime

Ingredients
- 18 Limes, Ripe
- 550g Caster Sugar

Method

1. Wash and dry 18 ripe limes to ensure that the skins are clean.
2. Remove the peel from the limes, without taking off the bitter white pith.
3. Set the lime peel aside.
4. Chop all of the limes in half and juice them all in a large mixing bowl.
5. Add 550g of caster sugar to the lime juice. Stir the ingredients together until all of the sugar has dissolved.
6. Crush the lime peels into the juice.
7. Stir the ingredients well and cover.
8. Place the lime juice in the refrigerator for 24 hours.
9. Place a sieve over a large clean bowl.
10. Strain the cordial by pouring it into the sieve. Leave the pulp to drip until all of the liquid has been collected.
11. Transfer the cordial into sterilised bottles or jars and seal.
12. Chill in the refrigerator for another 24 hours.
13. Serve diluted with cold or hot water.

*Top Tip

You can substitute the water and dilute the lime cordial with soda. Once you have opened the cordial, store in the refrigerator.

Lemon

Ingredients
- 8-10 Lemons, Unwaxed
- 650g Granulated Sugar
- Water

Method

1. Wash and dry 8-10 lemons to ensure that all of the skins are clean.
2. Remove the peel from the lemons, without taking off the bitter white pith.
3. Set the lemon peel aside.
4. Fill a large saucepan ¾ full with cold water and place over a medium/high heat. Bring the water to the boil.
5. Add the lemons to the boiling hot water and leave for 2-3 minutes.
6. Remove the lemons from the water and reserve lemon infused water.
7. Juice the lemons in a large bowl or in a jug.
8. Place 650g of granulated sugar in a medium sized saucepan and add the lemon zest and 500ml of lemon infused water.
9. Place the saucepan over a medium heat until all of the sugar has dissolved. Bring to a boil.
10. Add a further 500ml of lemon juice and bring to boiling point. Remove the saucepan from the heat.
11. Place the sieve over a large clean mixing bowl.
12. Strain the cordial by pouring it into the sieve. Leave the pulp to drip until all of the liquid has been collected.
13. Transfer the cordial into sterilised bottles or jars and seal.

14. Chill in the refrigerator for another 24 hours.
15. Serve diluted with water.

*Top Tip

You can substitute the water and dilute the lemon cordial with soda. Once you have opened the cordial, store in the refrigerator for up to 4 months.

Apple & Blackberry

Ingredients

- 1kg Apples

- 500g Blackberries

- 1 Lemon Juice

- Water

- 400g-800g Granulated Sugar

- A Pinch of Salt

Method

1. Wash 1kg of apples and roughly chop them into small wedges, removing any bruised bits.
2. Remove any stalks from the blackberries and any tatty pieces.
3. Place the blackberries in a bowl of fresh clean water and sprinkle them with a pinch of salt.
4. Rinse the blackberries well.
5. Add the apples and the blackberries to a large saucepan and cover ½ of the fruit with fresh cold water.
6. Place the saucepan over a low/medium heat, slowly bringing to a boil. Simmer for 15 minutes, until all of the fruit is soft.
7. Add the lemon juice to the saucepan.
8. Pour the fruit into a jelly bag, leaving it to drip into a bowl overnight.

9. Measure how much fruit juice you have extracted the next day, before pouring it into a large saucepan.
10. Add 400g of granulated sugar for each 500ml of fruit juice.
11. Place the saucepan over a low heat and gently heat the fruit juice, stirring occasionally. Make sure all of the sugar has dissolved before slowly bringing the liquid to a boil.
12. Boil for a further 5 minutes.
13. Strain the cordial by pouring it into the sieve. Leave the pulp to drip until all of the liquid has been collected.
14. Transfer the cordial into sterilised bottles or jars and seal.
15. Chill in the refrigerator for another 24 hours.
16. Serve diluted with water.

*Top Tip

You can substitute the water and dilute the apple and blackberry cordial with soda or prosecco. Once you have opened the cordial, store in the refrigerator.

Orange

Ingredients
- 8 Oranges
- Orange Zest
- 600ml Water
- 500g Granulated Sugar
- 15g Citric Acid

Method

1. Peel 4 oranges and remove as much of the white pith as you can from each of the oranges.
2. Place the orange segments in a large saucepan and add 500g of granulated sugar and 600ml of cold fresh water. Place the saucepan over a medium heat until all of the sugar has dissolved.
3. Bring to the boil.
4. Reduce the heat and simmer for 10-15 minutes.
5. Juice four oranges.
6. Remove the saucepan from the heat and add in the orange juice and 15g of citric acid. Stir the ingredients well and leave to cool for 2-3 hours.
7. Transfer the cordial into sterilised bottles or jars and seal.
8. Chill in the refrigerator for another 24 hours.
9. Serve diluted with water.

*Top Tip

You can substitute the water and dilute the orange cordial with soda or prosecco. Once you have opened the cordial, store in the refrigerator.

Mocktails

Tropical Apple Fizz

Ingredients
- 150ml of Apple Juice
- 3-4 Strips of Orange Peel
- 1 Tablespoon of Honey
- 1 Cinnamon Stick
- 3 Cloves

Method

1. Pour 150ml of apple juice into a saucepan and place over a medium heat.
2. Add 3-4 strips of orange peel to the apple juice and simmer.
3. Place the cinnamon stick in the saucepan along with 3 cloves.
4. Add one tablespoon of honey to sweeten.
5. Simmer the ingredients for a further 8-10 minutes before removing the saucepan from the heat.
6. The drink is ready to serve.

*Top Tip

Pour the drink into small tea glasses. Garnish each drink with a cinnamon stick and some orange peel.

Virgin Mary

Ingredients
- 150ml of Tomato Juice
- ½ Lemon (Juice only)
- 3 Dashes of Tabasco Sauce
- Pinch of Salt
- Pinch of Ground Black Pepper
- 6 Dashes of Worcestershire sauce
- 2 Ice Cubes

Garnish
- 1 Lemon Segment
- 1 Celery stick

Method

1. Place the 2 ice cubes in a tall glass or in a jug.
2. Pour 150ml of tomato juice into the glass over the ice cubes.
3. Add in ½ of lemon juice to the glass.
4. Add 3 dashes of Tabasco sauce and 6 dashes of Worcestershire sauce to the ingredients.
5. Sprinkle a pinch of salt and a pinch of ground black pepper into the glass and stir well.
6. The drink is ready to serve.
7. To garnish add one lemon segment and a stick of celery to each of the drinks.
8. The drink is ready to serve.

Cranberry Cocktail

Ingredients
- 85ml Red Cranberry Juice
- 85ml of Apple Juice
- 2 Tablespoons of Honey
- 2 Ice Cubes

Garnish
- A cherry

Method

1. Place the 2 ice cubes in a tall glass or in a jug.
2. Pour 85ml of red cranberry juice into the glass over the ice cubes.
3. Pour in 85ml of apple juice into the glass and mix together with the cranberry juice.
4. Stir in 2 tablespoons of honey.
5. To garnish add a cherry to each of the drinks.
6. The drink is ready to serve.

Shirley Temple

Ingredients
- 120ml Ginger Ale
- 30ml Grenadine
- 30ml Lime Juice
- 1 Slice of Orange
- 1 Maraschino Cherry
- Ice Cubes

Method

1. Place some ice cubes in a tall highball glass.
2. Pour 120ml of ginger ale, 30ml of grenadine and 30ml of lime juice in the highball glass over the ice cubes.
3. Garnish the drink with a slice of fresh orange and a maraschino cherry.
4. The drink is ready to serve.

*Top Tip

The grenadine will sink to the bottom of the glass and slowly rise to the top as you drink the cocktail.

Mojito

Ingredients

- 120ml Lemonade
- 60ml Apple Juice
- 1 Teaspoon Brown Sugar
- 1 Lime Juice
- 8 Sprigs of Mint
- Ice Cubes, Crushed

Method

1. Place the crushed ice cubes in a tall highball glass.
2. In a small bowl mash 1 teaspoon of brown sugar together with 4 sprigs of mint.
3. Add 20ml of the apple juice to the sugar.
4. Add the sugar mixture to the highball glass pouring over the crushed ice cubes.
5. Pour in the rest of the apple juice, and 120ml of lemonade.
6. Cut the lime in half and squeeze one-half of the lime juice into the glass.
7. Cut the other half of lime into 2 wedges and add to the glass.
8. Garnish with 4 sprigs of mint.
9. Stir the cocktail.
10. The drink is ready to serve.

Cosmopolitan

Ingredients

- 30ml Cranberry Juice
- 30ml Orange Juice, Fresh
- 30ml Lemon Juice, Fresh
- 30ml Lime Juice, Fresh
- Orange Zest
- Ice Cubes

Method

1. Pour 30ml Cranberry Juice, 30ml fresh orange juice, 30ml lime juice and 30ml of lemon juice into a cocktail shaker.
2. Add in some ice cubes and shake the cocktail shaker for 30-60 seconds.
3. Pour the cosmopolitan out into a clean martini glass.
4. Garnish with some orange zest.
5. The drink is ready to serve.

Sex on the Beach

Ingredients
- 60ml Cranberry Juice
- 60ml Orange Juice
- 30g Peach Nectar
- 1 Tablespoon of Grenadine
- 1 Pineapple Wedge
- Ice Cubes

Method

1. Pour 60ml of cranberry juice and 60ml of orange juice into either a jug or a tall glass.
2. Add 30g of peach nectar to the liquid and give it a quick stir.
3. Add some ice cubes to a tall highball glass.
4. Pour the drink into the highball glass over the ice cubes.
5. Add 1 tablespoon of grenadine to the drink.
6. Garnish with a pineapple wedge.
7. The drink is ready to serve.

*Top Tip

The grenadine will sink to the bottom of the glass and slowly rise to the top as you drink the cocktail. You can garnish your drink with a slice of orange instead of a pineapple wedge.

Strawberry Daiquiri

Ingredients
- 350g Strawberries, Frozen
- 1 Can of Pineapple Chunks in Juice
- 2 Tablespoons Fine Sugar
- 2 Limes, Juice
- 4 Fresh Strawberries
- Ice Cubes

Method

1. Empty 1 can of pineapple chunks into a blender.
2. Add in 350g of frozen strawberries to the blender, along with 2 tablespoons of fine sugar and the juice of 2 limes.
3. Blitz the blender for 1-2 minutes or until the ingredients turn smooth.
4. Pour the drink out into a cocktail glass.
5. Garnish with 4 fresh strawberries.
6. The drink is ready to serve.

Pina Colada

Ingredients

- 60ml Pineapple Juice, Unsweetened
- 30ml Cream of Coconut
- 1 Pineapple Wedge
- 1 Maraschino Cherry
- Ice Cubes

Method

1. Pour 60ml of unsweetened pineapple juice into a blender and add 30ml cream of coconut.
2. Add some ice cubes to the blender and blitz for 1-2 minutes, or until the texture of the drink turns thick.
3. Pour the drink out into a tall highball glass.
4. Garnish with a pineapple wedge and a maraschino cherry.

Tequila Sunrise

Ingredients

- 120ml Orange Juice
- 20ml Grenadine
- 1 Slice of Orange
- Ice Cubes

Method

1. Fill half of a tall highball glass with ice cubes.
2. Pour 120ml of orange juice into the glass over the ice cubes.
3. Slowly add in 20ml grenadine to the orange juice.
4. Garnish with a slice of orange.
5. The drink is ready to serve.

*Top Tip

The grenadine will sink to the bottom of the glass and slowly rise to the top as you drink the cocktail.

BIBLIOGRAPHY

Cross. F. L and Livingstone E A, ed
Oxford Dictionary of the Christian Church
Oxford University Press, 1997

NHS
Birth to Five
Crown 2009

NHS
The Pregnancy Book
The Department of Health
Crown 2009

National Childbirth Trust
NCT Pregnancy for parents by parents
The Department of Health
Collins 2000